Kausthub Des...
THE YOGA OF THE YOGI

Dr. Kausthub Desikachar, a son and student of T.K.V. Desikachar, began studying yoga when he was nine years old. After receiving a dual master's degree, he committed himself to becoming a full-time student and teacher of yoga. He recently completed doctoral studies at the University of Madras, where his topic of research was the effect of individualized yoga training on quality of life.

Kausthub is the cofounder of the Krishnamacharya Healing and Yoga Foundation (KHYF) and the chief strategic consultant to the Krishnamacharya Yoga Mandiram (KYM), where he is also a senior teacher and yoga therapy consultant. He is a patron of the British Wheel of Yoga, an adviser to the International Association of Yoga Therapists, and the founder of KYM-Mitra, a philanthropic organization that takes yoga to the differently abled and socially underprivileged.

Kausthub has written many books on yoga, including a biography of his grandfather the great yogi T. Krishnamacharya. He is also an accomplished photographer and poet and has published books in these areas as well.

THE YOGA OF THE YOGI

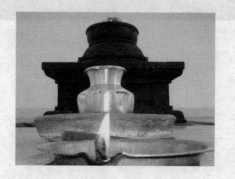

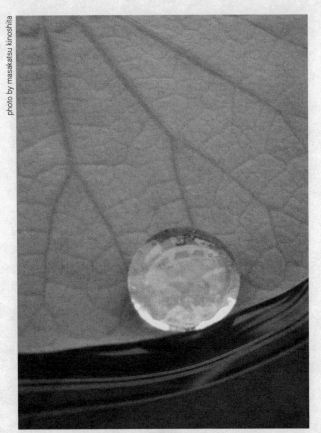

Water drop on lotus leaf.

THE YOGA OF THE YOGI

The Legacy of T. Krishnamacharya

Dr. Kausthub Desikachar

North Point Press
A division of Farrar, Straus and Giroux
New York

North Point Press
A division of Farrar, Straus and Giroux
18 West 18th Street, New York 10011

Copyright © 2005 by Kausthub Desikachar
Distributed in Canada by D&M Publishers, Inc.
Printed in India by Manipal Technologies Ltd
Originally published in 2005 by Krishnamacharya Yoga Mandiram, Chennai, India
Published in 2011 by North Point Press
First American edition, 2011

The photographs on the following pages are © Krishnamacharya Healing & Yoga Foundation: 2, 6, 20, 22, 33, 34, 37, 40, 47, 54–55, 56, 59, 68, 70, 76, 80, 82–83, 84, 86, 89, 90, 92, 94, 96, 98, 108, 118, 122, 147, 153, 162, 170, 174, 176, 178, 192, 206, 216, and 220.

Library of Congress Cataloging-in-Publication Data

Desikachar, Kausthub.
    The yoga of the yogi : the legacy of T. Krishnamacharya / Kausthub Desikachar.
        p.   cm.
    ISBN 978-0-86547-753-7 (pbk.)
    1. Krishnamacharya, T., b. 1888.   2. Yogis—India—Biography.   3. Yoga.   I. Krishnamacharya Yoga Mandiram (Madras, India).   II. Title.

    BL1175.K723D463 2011
    294.5092—dc23
    [B]

                                                                                            2011016107

Designed by Kausthub Desikachar
Editorial assistance by Elizabeth Bragdon and Scott Rennie

www.fsgbooks.com

10 9 8 7 6 5 4 3 2 1

dedicated to

namagiriamma	my grandmother
menaka desikachar	my mother
mekhala desikachar	my sister
lakshmi kausthub	my wife
sraddha kausthub	my daughter
piluca enriquez	my best friend

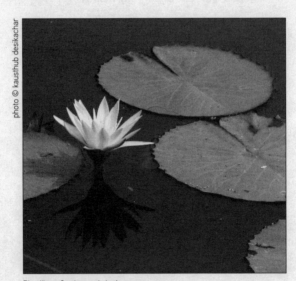

Blue lily, reflection, and shadow.

Acknowledgements

Many things came together during this project. It has not been an easy task to write the story of *yogacarya* T Krishnamacharya. There is so much we do not know about him, and at the same time, there is so much to say about what we do know. When you are working on a project like this, you either need a lot of luck or a lot of help. In my case, I had both. At every turn, I found myself running into the people I wanted to interview for this book or stumbling across photos to bring life to its pages. Friends generously contributed rare video footage that helped me enormously in my research. The entire project turned out to be a team effort, and I am very grateful to each and every member of this amazing team.

There are several people I would like to thank individually, starting with my father and teacher, TKV Desikachar. Not only did he ignite the spark of yoga in me, he also motivated me to tackle this project. I am grateful for his teaching, which revealed to me the magnitude and depth of yoga and the revolutionary accomplishments of Krishnamacharya. His constant encouragement (and all those cups of coffee he made for me) kept me going.

I would like to offer a special thanks to Mala Srivatsan for writing the first biography of Krishnamacharya, *Sri T Krishnamacharya: The Purnacarya*, in 1997. This book was one of my main inspirations.

A number of people helped with this project by contributing essays, anecdotes, photos, cookies, and warm words of encouragement. They include Pattabhi Jois, BKS Iyengar, Yvonne Millerand, MV Murugappan, MM Murugappan, TV Ananthanarayanan, AV Balasubramaniam, Mala Srivatsan, U Suresh Rao, Dr. B Ramamurthy, Prasanth Iyengar, S Sridharan, Lynn Carole Milich, Steve Annandale, Karina Friej, Barbara Brian, Sharath Rangaswamy, Eddie Stern, Larry Payne, Professor William Skelton, Frans Moors, Professor Varadachari, Professor Krishnamurthy Sastrigal, Maniam Selvam, Becky Gelatt, Amy Wheeler, and George Mantoan. I would also like to thank the entire staff and teachers of Krishnamacharya Yoga Mandiram, especially my secretary Jayanthi Sudhakar and the publications team: Asha Tilak, Raman Pillai, Nrthya Jagannathan, Lara Abhisheikh, and Ramakrishnan.

Many others contributed stories and shared their experiences with Krishnamacharya, but for personal reasons, they asked to remain anonymous. This is why some names used in this biography have been changed, while the names of others who provided me with information were not mentioned at all. My thanks to these contributors as well.

A very special thanks goes to my friends Todd Stellfox, Chase Bossart, Masakatsu Kinoshita, Hanna Persson, and Juan Pablo Martin. They understood my immersion in this project and forgave me for not being able to give them my complete attention while they were here in Chennai.

Words are not enough to express my gratitude to Liz and Scott, who offered invaluable editorial assistance on this book. They read the book again and again, refining the language, adjusting the placement of paragraphs, and just when I needed it, inspiring me to keep going.

I also have to thank Steve Jobs for inventing the Apple Macintosh, the Google founders for developing the most amazing search engine, and Adobe for creating Photoshop, InDesign, and Acrobat—all of which have been invaluable in making this project work.

This acknowledgement would not be complete without thanking my family—TKV Desikachar and Menaka Desikachar (my parents), Bhushan (my brother), Mekhala (my sister), Lakshmi (my wife), Sraddha (my daughter), and Tulsi (our dog).

Dr. Kausthub Desikachar

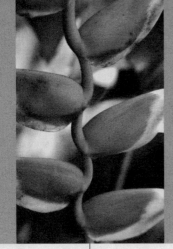

Contents

THE YOGA OF THE YOGI

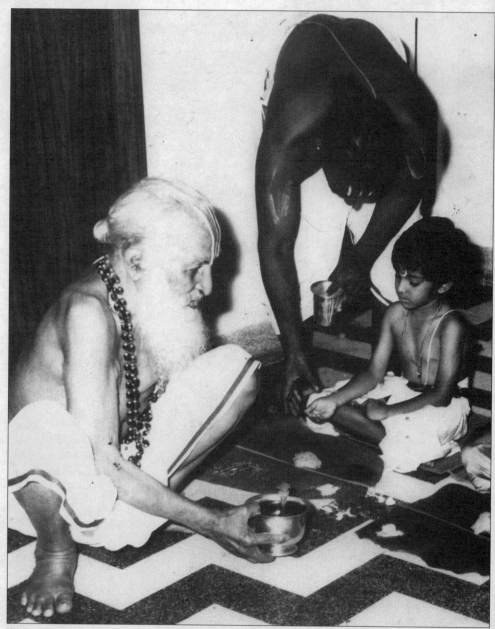

Krishnamacharya initiating Kausthub Desikachar at his sacred thread ceremony.

Prologue

A few months ago, I traveled to Tucson, Arizona, to teach a workshop on Yoga Therapy. A nice mix of people from around the country were gathered together that first morning of the workshop in a bright, friendly space filled with the smell of incense. There were young people and elderly people, healthy people as well as people with health concerns. As is my habit, I asked each person to introduce themselves to the group and tell us a bit about their background and the reason why they had come to this workshop.

Finally, it was the turn of an elderly lady in the front row to speak. I guessed her to be in her late eighties. She was sitting up very tall, and her eyes were clear, bright, and calm. She was smiling kindly. I was very impressed with her already, and when she began speaking, my heart melted at her words.

"I am Virginia Hill," she said. "I was a student of *Mataji* Indra Devi for many years, and I have come to meet you, the grandson of my teacher's teacher."

It was a humbling moment for me. I was overwhelmed that such an elderly lady had come all the way to this workshop to meet the grandson of her teacher's teacher. Such reverence for one's teacher and for the teachings is rare today. When I spoke with Virginia later, she told me how highly *Mataji* Indra Devi had spoken about her yoga teacher, Krishnamacharya, and this was the main reason she had come to meet me.

I was both overjoyed and terrified at the lady's words. I was overjoyed for many reasons: for being born into such a distinguished family and for being a student of yoga. Above all, I was overjoyed to meet this woman, the student of one of my grandfather's most devoted students.

And I was terrified, because at that moment I realized what an enormous responsibility I had, not just as a yoga teacher, but as a representative of two great masters—my grandfather, Tirumalai Krishnamacharya, and my father, TKV Desikachar. But as I thought about all of this and recalled the respect Virginia had offered me and the respect she had shown for the teaching tradition, I felt more confident and comfortable.

When I was younger, I was not interested in yoga. Probably, I was going through a bit of teenage rebellion. I wanted to do something different, something no one else in my family was doing. But my family's influence on me was strong, although very subtle. They never tried to force me to take part in their work, but I always knew the door to the world of yoga was open to me, if I chose to enter. Eventually, I decided on my own to look more carefully at what my family was offering me. Before long, I was a dedicated yoga student.

I have been fortunate to receive the teachings of yoga at home from my father, who is also my teacher. What a blessing to have this great teacher, who lives in my home, who is always close at hand. I never had to travel thousands of miles to learn, or work hard and save money to travel to a foreign land to pursue my practice. Nor did I have to make great sacrifices along the way. I was fortunate to have all the resources I needed right in my own backyard.

For this reason, I took it as my *dharma* (duty) to travel far away from my home and share with others what I have received from my teacher. My travels have taken me to almost every corner of the world. Along the way, I have met many people who share my passion for yoga, for whom its teachings are precious, just as they are to me. These are the people who inspire me every day to be a better student and a better teacher of yoga.

My travels have also opened my eyes to the confusion and discord that exists in the yoga community today.

"You have been talking so much about Patanjali. What is it, and how do you do that pose?"

I was teaching at a seminar in New Zealand, and it was the third day of our five-day session. The lady who asked me this question had been teaching yoga for ten years, yet she had no idea who Patanjali was. In her confusion, she had decided I must have been talking those three days about a posture. This was a shock to me. At that time, I thought every yoga teacher and yoga student knew of Patanjali, one of yoga's greatest teachers and author of the classic text, the *Yoga Sutra*.

On another journey that took me to New York, I was seated in a restaurant with some friends who were students and teachers of yoga. They had all learned yoga from different teachers, and so their practices differed considerably. When one of my friends ordered chicken for his lunch, two others pounced on him.

"How can you eat meat?" they demanded. "We are yoga teachers. We are supposed to be vegetarians."

When I asked them to elaborate on this theory that all yoga teachers must be vegetarians, they began to argue heatedly, justifying their position based on the concept of *ahimsa* (non-violence).

After they had quieted down a bit, I asked them, "If *ahimsa* is truly your underlying reason for choosing to be a vegetarian, why are you being so violent towards this man? Is your behavior to him not contrary to *ahimsa*?" I pressed on. "If all yoga practitioners are supposed to be vegetarians, what about people who live in places where it is difficult to find vegetarian food all year around? Places like Northern Russia, north of Canada, north of Sweden, etc. Are the people who live in these places not allowed to practice yoga?" This got them thinking.

On a recent flight to London from California, I was seated next to an outgoing elderly lady. Before long, I knew the history of her life and why she was traveling to England. After some time had passed, she seemed to realize that she had told me a great deal about herself, but knew nothing of me. So she turned the tables. "What do you do? Tell me about youself," she said.

4

When I told her that I was a yoga teacher, she immediately said, "So you went to California to learn yoga, right? I hear that it's the Mecca of yoga."

I smiled and told her that California is indeed a very popular place for yoga, but I had not gone there to learn, I had gone there to teach.

She was very surprised. "Are you telling me that a normal person like you can do yoga?"

Now it was my turn to be surprised. When I asked her to explain, she told me that she had always thought yoga was meant only for young, beautiful, flexible people. "This is why I never tried yoga, because I am not young and flexible. I can't think of myself in those strange poses," she said.

For the rest of our flight, I talked to this lady about yoga, and how it is open to everyone, regardless of age, flexibility level, or beauty. However, I was thinking as I explained all this to her, that her view was probably justified. Most yoga magazines, books, and videos showcase only the most beautiful people gifted with the most flexible, flawless bodies performing elegant poses against the most beautiful backdrops. While this presentation appeals to people on a few levels, playing up sex appeal and physical perfection against a background of serenity or natural beauty, it does not communicate the right message about yoga.

This is ironic, considering that most of the ancient yoga masters were not considered the most beautiful people, at least on the outside. For example, Veda Vyasa, a great *yogi* and saint, is actually considered one of the ugliest, as well. *Yogis* lived simple lives, typically in the mountains, and they did not care much about how they looked. Instead of focusing on outward appearance, they worked on refining the subtler aspects of human behavior, like their own attitudes and perceptions. They were not trying to sell anything, and they were not trying to buy anything. They practiced yoga, they taught yoga, and they lived their lives according to the teachings of yoga. To do this, they needed very little.

On a different journey, this one to Brazil, I was invited to attend a football match. Being a sports lover, I readily agreed. I assumed that I would be enjoying a match between two of the local football teams, until we pulled into a park instead of a stadium. Moments later, I found myself watching a football match between *Iyengar Yogis* and *Astanga Vinyasa Yogis*.

Intense rivalry is common in the sports world, but I had never seen anything quite like this. Players on both sides were aggressive and angry. They swore at each other frequently, and a fistfight nearly broke out at the end of the game.

Later, when I met with the team captains independently, I asked each one why the game had been so aggressive. They each gave me the same reply—the other team was "enemy camp."

Startled by this, I probed further. Did they know that both Mr. Iyengar and Mr. Pattabhi Jois (who are considered the pioneers of *Iyengar Yoga* and *Astanga Vinyasa Yoga*) had the same teacher?

"It can't be the same teacher," I heard from one. "They teach so differently."

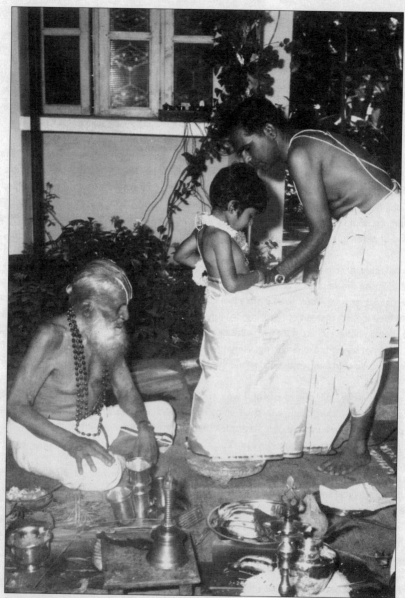

Desikachar helping Kausthub during his sacred thread ceremony. Krishnamacharya looks on.

"What we do is so different from the other camp," said the other.

These incidents occurred at different times and in different places over the course of my travels, but they all pointed me towards the same conclusion: there is a need to clarify many issues about yoga for this generation of students and teachers. There are serious students of yoga who do not know who Patanjali is or what the *Yoga Sutra* is. Most yoga students can recognize the names of four of the great yoga masters of this century—BKS Iyengar, Indra Devi, Pattabhi Jois, and TKV Desikachar—but they do not know that these masters share the same great teacher, **Tirumalai Krishnamacharya.**

I realized that by sharing the life of Krishnamacharya with a wider audience, I could help answer questions and bring clarification to some of the misunderstanding I have encountered in my work and travels. This book does not pretend to provide all of the answers to all of the questions, but I have attempted to address what I see as the core issues.

Also, rather than write a chronological biography, I sought to write a book that explores Krishnamacharya's life through the prism of his teachings. For this reason, not all events from his life are included here. At the same time, I believe everything important to understanding Krishnamacharya the *Pratinidhi* (torch bearer of the teachings) has been included. Hopefully, this book will inspire readers to delve more deeply into the teachings of yoga and the work of one of its greatest masters, Tirumalai Krishnamacharya.

My intention as the writer of this book is to let Krishnamacharya's actions, his accomplishments, the choices he made, and the way he lived his life speak for themselves. As a dedicated student and teacher of yoga, I believe it is important for anyone who is serious about yoga to know who Krishnamacharya was and to connect with his teachings.

Fernando Pages Ruiz put it best, perhaps, in an article entitled "The Legacy of Krishnamacharya," (*Yoga Journal*, May/June 2001):

"You may never have heard of him, but Tirumalai Krishnamacharya influenced or perhaps even invented your yoga. Whether you practice the dynamic series of Pattabhi Jois, the refined alignments of BKS Iyengar, the classical postures of Indra Devi, or the customized *vinyasa* [of Desikachar], your practice stems from one source: a five-foot, two-inch Brahmin born more than one hundred years ago in a small South Indian village."

Enjoy the journey.

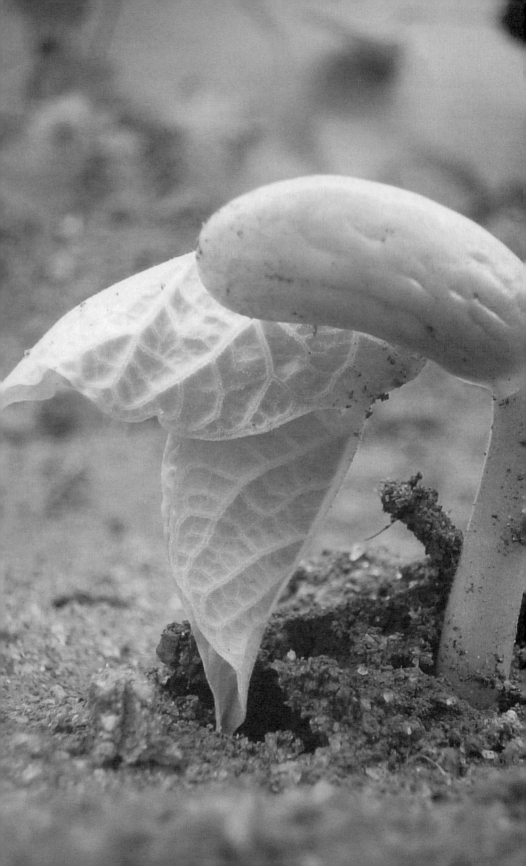

Chapter Zero

From Birth to Rebirth
yoga's long journey

the only sure thing is change.

"India is shining!" shouted recent billboards in Delhi, Mumbai, Chennai, and across the country

India has always been a crossroads of many worlds, a shining place. But today, it is a different India that shines. People all over the world are watching this ancient country with renewed interest. The computer revolution is changing the business landscape at an incredible rate, increasing the efficiency of India's corporate enterprises and government agencies. Pharmaceutical industries are producing high-quality drugs at a fraction of the cost of many modern countries, making expensive medicines more accessible to poorer nations. All over the country, industry is booming and national pride is on the rise. Despite the persistence of internal social and political challenges, India is well on its way to becoming a modern nation. It is not yet clear what gifts this new, modern India will bring to the world, but ancient India brought many gifts to humanity.

For centuries, people have been drawn to India as a land of many mysteries. India attracted invaders who coveted its land, sacred masters seeking to further their spiritual horizons, and merchants hoping to secure its resources for trade. From the digit zero, which revolutionized mathematics, to Mahatma Gandhi, who showed the world how a war could be won with love and peace; from New Delhi to New York; from the esoteric to the mundane, karma to curry, bollywood to bangra, the world has long been fascinated by all things Indian.

And today, the world is fascinated with yoga.

Once the realm of sacred masters in the Himalayas and spiritual ascetics, yoga is now practiced by people of every shape, size, and gender in every corner of the globe. And many of them want to know more about this ancient discipline.

Why was yoga invented? Who created it? What are its basic principles? What are its tools, and how can they be used? Are these poses that I do with my body truly yoga? And if this is all yoga is, then what is the difference between a *yogi* and a gymnast?

We can only imagine what life must have been like thousands of years ago when people first began practicing yoga. There were no cars, trains, or planes to take people from one place to another. If you wanted to go somewhere, you walked or ran. None of our modern means of communication existed. There were no telephones (mobile or otherwise), no postal service, and certainly, no e-mail. If people wanted to communicate with each other, they had to come together, face-to-face, and talk.

This was a time without pizza-delivery service, when the ingredients for every meal had to be hand-picked, hand-washed, and then cut and cooked by hand. The concept of pre-packaged food, a lifeless blob of indeterminate substances transformed after a few seconds in the microwave into a sticky toffee pudding, was as distant a dream as sending men to the moon. There were no dishwashers, no washing machines, and no bathtub to soak in after an exhausting day's work. If you wanted to wash anything, you needed a strong back and two strong hands, and hopefully, there was a clean water source nearby. If not, it meant only one thing—a very long walk.

It was in this physically demanding world that yoga originated. In other words, the first people to practice yoga did not need an exercise regimen. Everyday life provided them with more than enough opportunity to engage in physical activity. We need to keep this fact in mind as we consider the purpose for which yoga was conceived.

What our ancestors did share with us, if not our modern conveniences and sedentary lifestyle, was the urge to explore, not just the physical world, but the spiritual one, as well. *Who am I? Why am I here? What should I do? What are my responsibilities?* They were concerned with issues of the mind and soul, with the causes of psychological and spiritual suffering, or *duhkham*, as it is called in Sanskrit.

Eventually, the efforts of early Indian philosophers to find the solution to *duhkham* resulted in the founding of the various schools of Indian philosophy. Although the goal of each school was the same—to reach the spiritual core of the human being and eliminate *duhkham*—their paths were distinct. Of the countless philosophical schools that arose in India, there are six that came to be considered the most important, because they shared a common source, the *Vedas*.

The *Vedas* are a vast body of teachings believed to be the oldest source of knowledge in India. They are known as an *agama*, or a "definitive reference." No one knows who created the *Vedas*, when they were created, or even whether they were all composed by the same author. Only one thing is certain; they are considered the most sacred among all the Indian teachings. It is believed that almost all that is important to know has been discussed in the *Vedas*. In India, the *Vedas* are considered the absolute reference for any teachings or teacher.

Collectively, the six philosophical schools were known as the *Sat Darsanas*. *Sat*, meaning "six," and *Darsana*, meaning "philosophy" (coming from the root *drs*—to see, to understand). Yoga is one school among these *Sat Darsanas*. The other five schools are *Mimamsa*, *Nyaya*, *Vaisesikha*, *Samkhya*, and *Vedanta*. All six schools share the goal of removing *duhkham* through spiritual practice, but beyond this, yoga differs significantly from the others, especially in the way it approaches *duhkham*.

Mimamsa emphasizes the role of our actions and rituals in reducing *duhkham*. According to this school, if we perfect our actions, mundane and spiritual, we will never suffer.

Nyaya emphasizes logic and establishing cause-and-effect relationships between everything that is happening in the world. Everything happens because of a cause, including suffering. If we address the cause of *duhkham*, we can rid ourselves of it.

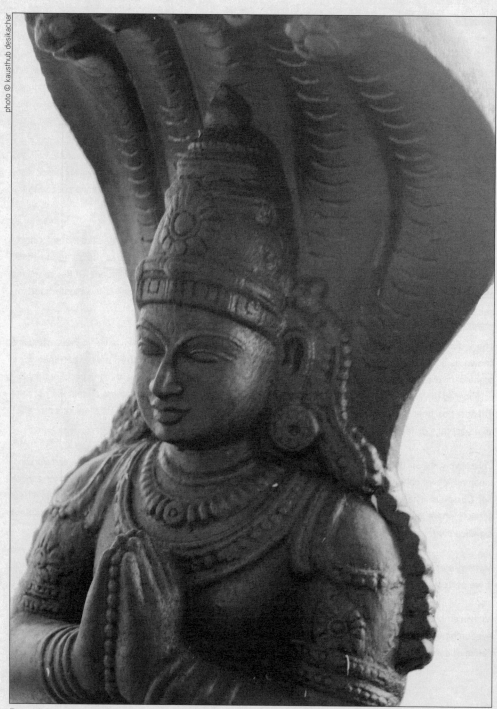

Patanjali, considered the father of yoga. He is also the author of the *Yoga Sutra*.

According to the teachings of *Vaisesikha*, everything in this world goes through a stage of evolution and dissolution, including our actions. If we understand this correctly, and act according to the right stage of our action's evolution, then we remain happy and avoid pain.

Samkhya says that life is a combination of two things: a part that is conscious (*purusa*) and a part that is not conscious (*prakrti*). While the consciousness is *purusa*, the body, mind, and senses are *prakrti*. *Prakrti* depends on *purusa* for existence. At the same time, the *purusa* needs the *prakrti* in order to function. This close link between the two is what allows life to proceed successfully. Sometimes, however, there is confusion over who is the master. Imagine, for example, if the horses thought they were in charge of directing the course of the carriage. When this happens there is a runaway carriage, and this can cause a lot of trouble. *Samkhya* helps clarify the roles of *purusa* and *prakrti*, so that we don't get into trouble.

Finally, *Vedanta* holds that religion is the cure for suffering. *Vedanta* became the foundation of what is now known as *Hinduism*.

To find out what yoga has to say about *duhkham*, we start with the *Yoga Sutra*, an ancient text of yoga teachings compiled by a great *yogi* called Patanjali. The *Yoga Sutra* is considered the definitive reference on yoga. *Yogis* revered this text to such a degree that disputes were often settled based solely on the content of the *Yoga Sutra*.

From the outset, Patanjali makes it very clear in the *Yoga Sutra* that yoga is more about dealing with the mind than anything else, including the physical body:

> **yogah citta vrtti nirodhah | Yoga Sutra I. 2**
>
> *yoga is to direct the mind on a chosen focus and maintain that focus without distraction*

Presented in a simple aphoristic style over four chapters, Patanjali's *Yoga Sutra* lays out the road map of yoga. The basic premise of Patanjali's teaching is that our human mind is both the source of and solution to our problems. If the mind is distracted or agitated, then we get into trouble. But if the mind is focused and calm, it helps us solve the problems we encounter in everyday life and leads us forward on the path towards our spiritual core. This is the simple essence of the teachings of yoga, and the reason why it was developed thousands of years ago.

But dealing with the mind is not a simple task. Before we can direct our mind, we must first develop an understanding of its workings and identify any obstacles that must be overcome. This takes considerable time, effort, and careful guidance, which the *Yoga Sutra* offers us.

Patanjali had a profound understanding of the way the human mind functions. He understood that the mind has many different dimensions and supports many different activities, states, and functions. He also understood the multitude of influences that affect the mind. These influences, in turn, affect the mind's character, functioning, and even its qualities.

Patanjali knew, for example, that the body influences the mind. If my body is tired or stressed, so is my mind. If my body is relaxed and calm, then my mind is relaxed and calm. He also understood the role of the breath in affecting the mind. When the breath is agitated, the mind becomes agitated. When the breath is smooth and steady, the mind is smooth and steady. Similarly, the food we eat, our lifestyle, the company we keep, our emotional state, etc., all of these things affect the mind.

The reverse is also true. If we influence our state of mind, other aspects of the human system are influenced in a similar manner. For example, if my mind is agitated, my breath is agitated. But if I then listen to some soothing music and calm my mind, the breath also becomes calm.

In essence, what Patanjali grasped was that all aspects of the human system—the physical aspect, the breath, the intellectual aspect, the personality, the emotions—are interrelated. And so he gifted us, through the teachings of yoga, with a wide range of tools to treat the needs of the entire human system holistically. For Patanjali, there was no such thing as a **"one-pill-cures-all"** approach. The yoga toolbox provides a wide range of tools, and they can be utilized based on the student's needs in an infinite number of combinations for health, healing, and spiritual evolution. These tools include conscious breathing regulation (*pranayama*), body positions (*asana*), dietary recommendations (*ahara niyama*), lifestyle recommendations (*vihara niyama*), social attitudes (*yama*), personal disciplines (*niyama*), meditation (*dhyanam*), visualizations (*bhavana*), sensory control (*pratyahara*), and more.

A few years ago I asked my father, who is also my teacher, "If I had to study just one text on yoga, what would you recommend?"

Without a moment's hesitation, he replied, "The *Yoga Sutra* of Patanjali." He added, "I too asked the same question of my teacher and got the same answer."

Of course, this does not mean that the other texts are not important, but since these texts base their teachings on the *Yoga Sutra*, it makes sense to concentrate more on the *agama* itself.

I believe that it was the same for many yoga masters throughout history. Naturally, these masters drew inspiration from the culture, lifestyle, and habits of their times in order to evolve teaching paradigms that fit the context of their lives and the lives of the people they worked with. This is why the teaching practices of the various yoga schools differ. However, what they all teach is still yoga, and at the end of the day, most still consider the *Yoga Sutra* their definitive guide.

For all of its promise and successes, yoga has not always enjoyed the popularity it does today. Time and time again, outside forces invaded India and sought to destroy the native culture and replace it with their own. But because of the spiritual strength of the teachings and of the great masters, this knowledge outlived the invaders. Over time, it helped to maintain the integrity of the Indian land and its wisdom. Of course, not everything survived the test of time, and India lost many great teaching traditions, but we are thankful for the wealth of knowledge that remains.

One of these cultural declines occurred in India at the beginning of the twentieth century. Many traditions, including yoga, were facing extinction as people looked to the rapidly modernizing and expanding West. Under British rule, Western medicine, the Western educational system, and Western values were promoted throughout India and slowly began to replace the existing native institutions. Yoga, among many other traditions, was dying. Few people were interested in its ancient teachings, and those who were did not have access to the most profound secrets. Yoga's teachings were at risk of being diluted, transformed into a dull handbook of physical exercises.

When we enter a tunnel, the darkness surrounds us, giving the impression that all is lost. But sooner or later, the light breaks through again. And so it was with yoga. This light came in the form of a man from South India. Over the course of a lifetime that spanned more than one hundred years, he would bring life back into the dying world of yoga and revolutionize its practice for a modern world.

Chapter One

A Boy Always Hungry
the torch is lit

when we are really thirsty, we will definitely find water.

In India, there are many different religious traditions, and each tradition worships a different God as the primordial Being. For example *Vaisnava* followers worship Lord *Visnu* as their only deity, while those belonging to the rival *Saiva* tradition worship Lord *Siva*, the dancing God.

In South India, the most popular religious school is *Sri Vaisnava Sampradayam*. Followers of this tradition worship Lord *Visnu*, along with his consort, Goddess *Laksmi*, as the primordial Supreme Beings. Those who practice *Sri Vaisnava Sampradayam* today owe the tradition's richness and longevity to a master called Nammalvar. Little is known about Nammalvar, but he was one the first masters of the tradition, establishing the *Sri Vaisnava Sampradayam* school with the help of some of his contemporaries. Together, they were known as *Alvars*.

Nammalvar was born into a family of hunters. The exact date of his birth is unknown. He was called Maran, which means "abnormal" or "different from others" (it was only later that he would be known as Nammalvar). His parents gave him this unusual name, because he did not cry at the time of his birth, or drink his mother's milk, or do many other things that normal children do.

One day, Maran's parents heard a voice tell them to leave the infant in the hollow of a tamarind tree. Believing this to be the voice of the Divine and that Maran must be destined for great things, the couple sought out the tamarind tree and left the child there. The tree became Maran's home.

Sixteen years later, a learned man named Madhurakavi was traveling through the north of India when a strong light suddenly appeared in the south. Every day, Madhurakavi would see this light glowing in the south, and he decided that God was directing him to find the source of the light. He turned south, and eventually, he arrived in a small village in South India called Alvar Tirunagari, in Tirunelveli district. Here, the shining light merged into the figure of a young man sitting quietly in the hollow of a tamarind tree. The young man appeared lost in meditation.

Madhurakavi tried to get the meditator's attention. He threw stones on the ground. He clapped loudly. He called the youth names. But the boy remained unmoved. Finally, Madhurakavi decided to ask the young man a question. "When the un-manifest takes birth in the manifest, what will it eat, and what will it do?"

The youth's eyes immediately lit up, and he answered promptly, "It will eat the manifest and remain in it."

Stunned by the boy's riddle-like, yet profound reply, the learned Madhurakavi prostrated himself before him (an unconventional act in those days, when the younger one was required to prostrate to the elder,) and declared that he, Madhurakavi, had finally found his teacher.

It was after this incident that Maran, the young man under the tamarind tree, became known as Nammalvar. The word *Nammalvar* has many meanings, including "the one who has come to lead us."

Over the next decade, Nammalvar's teachings, *Tiruviruttam, Tiruvasiriyam, Periya Tiruvantati*, and the classic *Tiruvaimozhi*, formed the foundation of *Sri Vaisnava Sampradayam*. The writings were devotional in nature, instructing students to love God in a sublime way.

Nammalvar lived only thirty-five years. Some believe that his short life span was the result of sickness. Others contend that his life ended early because he had fulfilled the mission entrusted to him.

Nammalvar's student, Madhurakavi, continued his master's work spreading the teachings of *Sri Vaisnava Sampradayam* to other *Alvars*, who would go on to do the same, in their turn. The collective works of Nammalvar and the *Alvars*, which set forth the entire *Sri Vaisnava* belief system, is called *Divya Prabandham*. The *Divya Prabandham* consists of four thousand verses in Tamil language, one of the most prominent and oldest languages in South India.

The turmoil of war and invasion would eventually take its toll on many of India's cultural traditions, including *Sri Vaisnava Sampradayam*, and by the ninth century, the teachings were in danger of being lost. It was during this troubled time that Nathamuni, one of the greatest *acaryas* (torch bearing masters) of *Sri Vaisnava Sampradayam*, was born.

Nathamuni was born in the year 823 AD to a pious family in the township of Viranarayanapuram, near Chidambaram (about three hours drive from modern day Chennai). He received a conventional education from his father, Iswara Bhatta, and learned music from his mother. He showed a deep interest in spiritual matters early on and mastered many of the great philosophies that were in vogue at the time. By the time he reached middle age, he had become a popular, highly respected teacher with his own following of students.

One day, Nathamuni came upon a group of mystics singing verses praising Lord *Visnu*. Enraptured by the mystics' magical chants, which he had never heard before, Nathamuni followed them. He asked the mystics what they were chanting, and if they would teach it to him. They told him that the verses were from Nammalvar's *Divya Prabandham*, and there were only ten of them. The other three thousand nine hundred and ninety verses had been lost.

However, one of the mystics told Nathamuni, he might obtain the lost verses if he traveled to the tamarind tree where Nammalvar was discovered and recited these ten verses tens of thousands of times.

Nathamuni promptly learned the ten verses, and when he had gathered enough resources, he traveled to the tamarind tree. Nathamuni sat in *Padmasana* in the hollow of the tree and began to recite the ten verses with great devotion. According to legend, Nammalvar appeared to Nathamuni during this meditation and helped him recover the three thousand nine hundred and ninety lost verses of the *Divya Prabandham*.

This vision and the gift of the lost verses established a strong link between Nammalvar and Nathamuni. Armed with the recovered verses, Nathamuni set out to revitalize the *Sri Vaisnava Sampradayam*. His

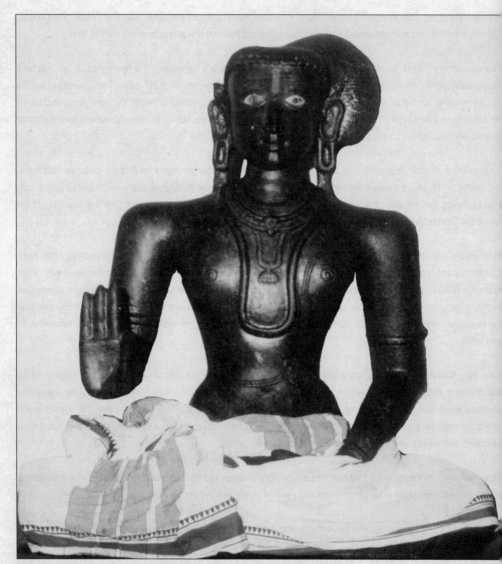

Nammalvar, one of the founding fathers of *Sri Vaisnava Sampradayam*.

passion for his mission was so intense that he quickly re-established the *Sri Vaisnava Sampradayam* and gathered a vast number of followers from all over South India to the tradition.

In addition to teaching the lost verses of the *Divya Prabandham*, Nathamuni also offered the teachings of his own texts, especially the *Nyaya Tattva* and *Yoga Rahasya*. He dedicated the rest of his life to spreading the message of *Sri Vaisnava Sampradayam* to ensure that it would never be lost again. Today, Nathamuni is worshipped in India as a God for having succeeded at a task that many believed was beyond a human being's abilities.

Nathamuni's accomplishments were not limited to the revival of *Sri Vaisnava Sampradayam*, he was also a master of many other teachings, including yoga. He composed a text called *Yoga Rahasya* (*Secrets of Yoga*), which elaborates on many important and practical yoga teachings found in the classical yoga texts. Few such texts exist, and for this reason, *Yoga Rahasya* is considered one of Nathamuni's most precious works. In it, he explains how to adapt yoga to different stages of life, the importance of yoga for women, especially pregnant women, and the role of yoga in healing, among many other topics. Ironically, the *Yoga Rahasya* was lost a few years after Nathamuni's death.

Many believed that the *Yoga Rahasya* was lost forever, including a man named Srinivasa Tatacarya and his wife, Ranganayakiamma, who lived in ninteenth-century Mucukundapuram, South India. The couple came from an illustrious family and could trace their heritage all the way back to Nathamuni himself.

On the 18th of November 1888, Ranganayakiamma gave birth to a boy, their first child. They named him Krishnamacharya, after Lord *Krsna*, one of the incarnations of Lord *Visnu*. Krishnamacharya was soon joined by two brothers, Narayana and Appalacarya, and three sisters: Alamelu, Tayamma, and Cudamani.

As a boy, Krishnamacharya was tutored by his father, a great scholar in his own right. Srinivasa Tatacarya supervised several students who studied the *Vedas* and many other religious texts in the traditional *gurukula* manner.

Under the *gurukula* system, the student lived in the house of the teacher learning everything that needed to be learned. Only when the teacher felt the student had completed his education was he allowed to leave the *gurukula*. It was in his father's *gurukula* that Krishnamacharya received his early education.

The *gurukula* system was a very personal and powerful system of education. The teacher and the student worked together one-on-one, and there were typically no more than twelve students in the *gurukula* at one time. This ensured quality time for each student and allowed the teacher to develop a clear picture of each student's strengths, weaknesses, and potential. Knowing his students so well, the teacher could teach each one in the manner most advantageous for that student. This close relationship that develops between students and teachers through the *gurukula* system is called *upadesa*. The word can be split into two parts: *upa* meaning "nearby," and *desa* meaning "place." Translated literally, it means the distance

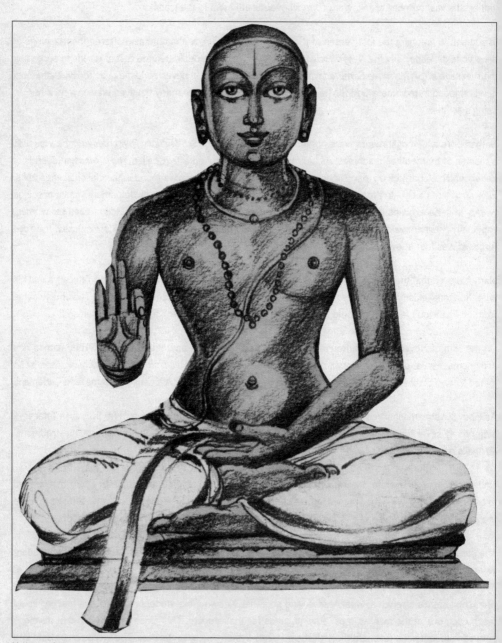

Nathamuni, the grand master, who revived *Sri Vaisnava Sampradayam*.

between teachers and students was quite short; they were close to each other, connected, even when the teaching was done.

In those days, teachers were extremely strict with their students. They valued the teachings above all else, so the regimen at the *gurukula* was not an easy one. Srinivasa Tatacarya woke his students at 2:00 a.m. to chant the *Vedas* and practice *yoga asanas*. The students had to repeat the *Vedic* chants from memory until they could recite them free of mistakes. They also had to learn all the sacred rites and procedures.

So it was Krishnamacharya's father, his first *guru* (teacher), who planted the seed of knowledge in him and guided and encouraged him in his quest for learning.

Krishnamacharya lost this precious guidance at the age of ten, when Srinivasa Tatacarya died. At the time, the Pontiff of the Parakala Math in Mysore City, the capital of the South Indian kingdom of Mysore, was Srinivasa Tatacarya's grandfather. The Math Center was as important to *Sri Vaisnava Sampradayam* as the Vatican is to Christianity. It was the hub of all the religious and spiritual activities that centered around the teachings of Nathamuni and Vedanta Desikacarya, a master of *Sri Vaisnava Sampradayam* and the center's founder. The center was responsible for education, initiation, and dissemination of the *Sri Vaisnava Sampradayam* teachings. It was convention in those days for the King of the land to have a spiritual teacher, and often this teacher was the Pontiff of the Parakala Math.

To facilitate the continuing education of Krishnamacharya and his siblings, the family shifted to Mysore, and Krishnamacharya enrolled as a pupil of the Math.

Under the watchful eye of his great-grandfather, and then his great-grandfather's successor, Sri Krsna Brahmatantra Swami, Krishnamacharya began learning *Vyakarana* (Sanskrit Grammar), *Vedanta*, and *Tarka* (Logic). Soon, he was proficient in a number of subjects and engaged himself in debates with the professors and visiting scholars. These exchanges ignited his hunger for wisdom, and, to quote his own words, "that was how I found out that there was so much more to learn."

At the age of sixteen, Krishnamacharya had a strange dream. In this dream, his ancestor Nathamuni directed him to go to Alvar Tirunagari, the same small town in the neighboring state of Tamilnadu where Madhurakavi discovered Nammalvar meditating in the hollow of the tamarind tree. This was also where Nathamuni later rediscovered the lost teachings of Nammalvar.

Krishnamacharya could not ignore the vision and the request of his ancestor, so he gathered together the necessary resources for his journey and set out, a boy of sixteen, on a mission to find the tamarind tree. In those days traveling was difficult and distances seemed much greater than they actually were. Mysore is about six hundred kilometers from Alvar Tirunagari, and Krishnamacharya did not have a motorcar or the money to buy train tickets, but he was not discouraged. He walked in the grueling heat of the sun, day after day. He slept under trees or at the *thinnai*, a kind of balcony built at the entrance of houses in those days, mainly for the purpose of providing travelers a place to sleep.

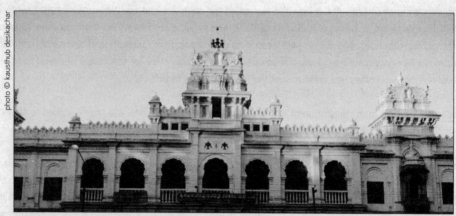

The front portion of the Parakala Math, Mysore, as it looks today.

When Krishnamacharya arrived at his destination, he encountered an old man seated under a tree. Krishnamacharya told the old man about his dream and asked him where he could find Nathamuni. The old man only moved his head, indicating a particular direction. Krishnamacharya walked in the direction the old man had shown him, and soon found himself standing in the middle of a mango grove by the side of the river, Tamraparani. Tired and hungry from his long, arduous journey, he fell unconscious.

In this state, a trance gripped him, and he found himself in the presence of three sages. He prostrated before them and told them of his dream and requested to be instructed in the *Yoga Rahasya*. Nathamuni, seated between the other two sages, began reciting the verses, and his voice was very musical. When the discourse was over, Krishnamacharya opened his eyes to find that there was no grove, and the three sages were gone. But he remembered every single one of the verses that Nathamuni had chanted.

Krishnamacharya ran back to tell the old man what had happened. The old man smiled and said, "You are very lucky to have received the *Yoga Rahasya*. Now go inside and offer your prayers to Lord *Visnu* to thank him for his benevolence."

Krishnamacharya ran into the temple that had been erected to Lord *Visnu* at this sacred site and offered his prayers. When he went back outside, the old man was gone. As Krishnamacharya stood there recalling the incident in the mango grove, it slowly dawned on him that the old man who had directed him to the grove and then to the temple resembled the sage who had recited the verses to him in his trance. It was only then that he realized that he had received the *Yoga Rahasya* from Nathamuni himself.

Later in his life, it became clear to Krishnamacharya that this incident had been a test of his commitment to yoga, as well as a directive from both Nammalvar and Nathamuni to spread the teachings of yoga. Just as Nammalvar and Nathamuni established the *Sri Vaisnava Sampradayam* and worked to ensure that the tradition remained strong and vibrant, Krishnamacharya would go on to revive the teachings of yoga and provide the yoga tradition with a strong, revitalized base from which to grow and spread.

As the product of a modern educational system grounded in science and rationalism, I was skeptical of this story. But when I visited this place, Alvar Tirunagari, my opinion changed.

It is a simple place. The town has not commercialized or exploited the temple at the site of the tamarind tree. The atmosphere is pure. There is a sense of stillness in the air.

My friends and I sat before the tamarind tree and did some chanting. After a while, a deep feeling was aroused within me. Normally I am restless and very active; always on the move. I have never spent more than ten minutes in any temple in India. But somehow I did not want to move from this place. Tears filled my eyes, and I did not know why. I could see that some of my friends were similarly affected. I noticed that the friends in our group who are usually very restless and aggressive were suddenly peaceful and calm. Two others, who had argued just before entering this place, embraced each other with great warmth. At this moment, I knew that this was no ordinary place.

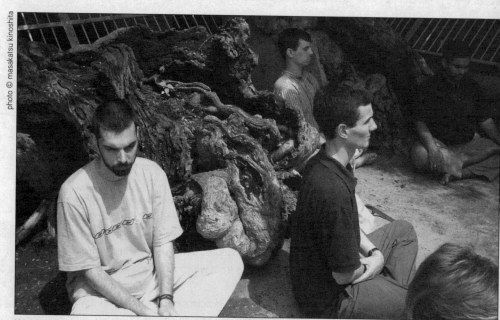

Kausthub Desikachar (right) and friends at the base of the tamarind tree, as it looks today.

Maturity dawned in me. I realized that what had happened to Nammalvar, Nathamuni, and Krishnamacharya at this holy place could not be just a fantasy. It was then that I decided to begin work on this biography.

As we mature spiritually, we begin to understand that things happen for a reason. And we also recognize that there is often some divine intervention that supports us and our mission when we least expect it. When the *Sri Vaisnava* tradition was declining and Nathamuni set out to revive it, he needed support to complete his task. Probably, this is why he received the *Divya Prabandham*.

Similarly, when yoga was facing its dark days in the early twentieth century, Krishnamacharya needed support to fulfill his mission and preserve the tradition of yoga. This may be the reason for the divine intervention that allowed him to recover the lost teachings of the *Yoga Rahasya*, which would become such an invaluable tool in his work.

Krishnamacharya's experience in Alvar Tirunagari clarified for him what his role would be in the world of yoga. He also knew that he would need help to revive this great Indian tradition. Knowledge of the *Yoga Rahasya* alone would not be enough, he would need a broad base of knowledge to work from, the very best of India's wisdom, in order to present yoga in a proper and just manner. Hungry to learn, he embarked on a journey—a quest—that would take him all over India.

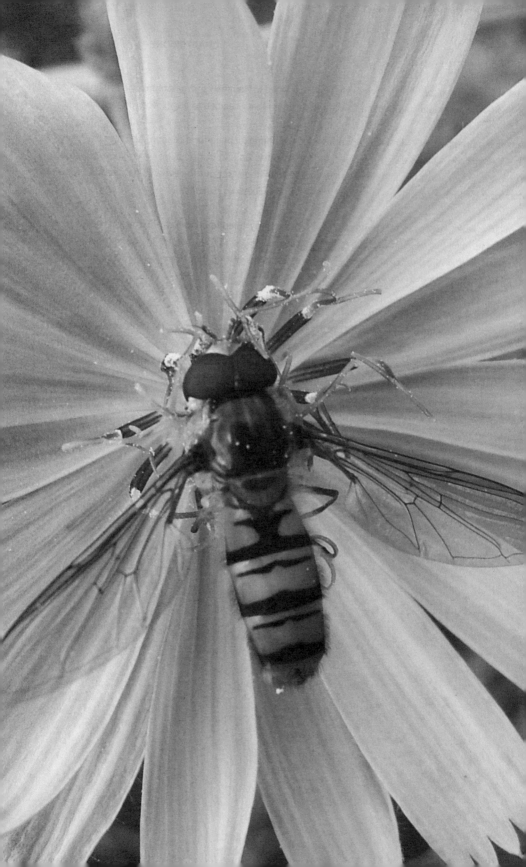

Chapter Two

Holistic Body, Holistic Outlook
the doctrine of yoga

a flower is not just how it appears,
but also how it smells, feels, and tastes.

"This is Steve," announced Barbara, my friend from Melbourne, Australia.

Steve was an energetic man in his thirties. He worked for an airline with a high-stress profile, but the stress and long hours had not stopped him from pursuing his passion for fly-fishing, hiking, and landscape gardening. He partied hard, drank a lot, and basically enjoyed his life. A very independent man, Steve prided himself on the fact that he was not dependent on others for anything. At times, this independence seemed more like stubbornness and even made some people feel uncomfortable around him, but none of this bothered Steve. He lived life by his own rules.

All of this changed one Wednesday. While working in Melbourne Airport, Steve blacked out and collapsed to the floor. He regained consciousness to find himself in a hospital unable to speak or move. Doctors informed him that he had suffered a massive stroke.

Steve was devastated. Because of the severe injury to his brain, he was now completely paralyzed on the left side of his body. He could no longer walk or move around, and he had lost the ability to speak. He was, essentially, bedridden. He could not return to work, he could not pursue his passions, and he couldn't go out and party with his friends. He had to come to grips with the fact that he was dependent on others for every little thing.

Steve explained to me how the stroke had affected him. "The whole left side of my body was affected. My leg and arm would not respond. The shock of losing muscle tone was even greater. Considering that it takes from birth to late childhood or early adulthood to really learn how to refine our movements, to lose that ability is a shock. I often think about the transition that a baby makes to walk. That's where I had to begin. I have had to learn all those fine motor skills again. I have had to go back and work on muscles that we take for granted as adults. The same with my balance. Without strength in my ankles, I simply don't have any balance. I have to place all my mind's energy into my ankle when I'm doing a balance, and at the same try not to lock my knee in the process. I lost my speech. I thought, 'Gosh!!! How am I going to communicate?' My sharp mind is a big part of who I am. Finding a way to express this was a priority for me. I had to relearn how to spell, write, and do mathematical calculations."

In a flash, everything that personified the old Steve was gone. Well, not quite everything. He was still very stubborn, which would turn out to be a blessing in disguise.

As part of his recovery, Steve worked with a physiotherapist to recover some of his muscle tone. An acupuncturist worked on bringing sensation back in his left side, and Steve also worked with a speech therapist. A doctor supervised the entire course of treatment.

During one of Steve's speech therapy sessions, the therapist told him, "You must do something to ensure that this does not happen to you again."

Steve took this advice very seriously and began thinking about what may have caused the stroke. He knew that the reason probably had a great deal to do with the stressful, intense pace of his work and life. Clearly, if he wanted to avoid another stroke in the future, he would have to reduce his stress level. Steve remembered hearing that yoga was good for reducing stress. His friend Valerie introduced him to a yoga teacher, Barbara Brian.

From their very first session together, Steve realized that Barbara's approach to healing was different from that of the other therapists and doctors. It was more unified, encompassing, and holistic.

Yoga teaches that the human system is a holistic unit comprised of several dimensions or levels. We are not just a physical body, our human system is much more complex than that. We have a breathing body that keeps us alive. We are made up of senses, which help us feel and perceive the world around us. We have a mind or intellect, which allows us to perceive and analyze things in a particular way. A philosopher will look at a situation in one way, for example, while a scientist will look at the same situation in an entirely different way.

We are also made up of different personality traits. For example, some of us are extroverted, others are introverted. And we have emotions. Holding an infant in our arms, we are immediately filled with inexplicable joy. When we are stuck in a traffic jam for a long time, we may begin to feel agitated and frustrated. Some people even become enraged. All of these feelings are a part of who we are.

These dimensions of the human system—the physical body, the breath, the mind, the personality, and the emotions—are deeply interconnected. As an example, if you enjoy holding a sleeping baby in your arms, continue to do so for a reasonable time, and you will begin to notice that your breathing changes and becomes calmer. Your senses, your physical body, your emotions, all come into play and affect your mind, your breath, and each other.

Imagine another scenario. I am just returning from a successful meditation retreat. I feel very calm as I drive my car home. I enter the highway and become stuck in a traffic jam, which seems to last forever. The longer the halt seems to be, the faster my breathing becomes. The body becomes restless, and soon I am bursting with anger. So we can see that these layers do not remain distinct from one another; they are interactive and interdependent.

Yoga, and almost every school of Indian thought, including the *Vedas*, accepts this holistic model of the human system. Patanjali speaks of it in depth in the *Yoga Sutra*. He says that when we suffer, our suffering may express itself through four kinds of symptoms: emotional suffering, pessimistic attitude, physiological changes in our body, and an irregular breathing pattern.

duhkha daurmanasya angamejayatva svasaprasvasah viksepa sahabhuvah |
Yoga Sutra I. 31

emotional disturbance, negative thinking, bodily reaction, and changes in breathing pattern are
the symptoms that accompany the agitated [person]

Sometimes these symptoms may manifest singly, while in some other situations, they manifest in combination. For example, we may have a mild fever (a physiological change), and that is all. But in another situation, I may have a fever and become extremely depressed about it. As a result, my breathing pattern may change, becoming heavy.

This is a very important point to understand. Patanjali does not view a person with suffering as someone with problems in the physical body only. Suffering, in any of its forms, is not a disease of the body alone or the mind alone or the emotions alone, because all of these dimensions of our human system are interconnected. Yoga understands and deals with the body as a holistic system. As therapists in yoga, we must learn to look at the human system in its fullest, richest expression, in its completeness and complexity, rather than as one flat dimension.

For example, sometimes people will come to me complaining of chronic neck pain. If I were to look at this problem as only a neck problem and continue to give exercises for the neck only, the treatment might or might not work. The cause of the neck pain may be stress, and for many people, stress does show up first in the neck.

But if we delve into the problem more deeply by looking into the person's lifestyle choices, for example, we may actually determine the source of the stress causing the neck pain. Once we address the source of stress directly and eliminate it, the neck pain will vanish automatically.

However, if we only treat the symptom (the neck pain), we may alleviate it, but the source of the pain will remain. This means the neck pain could reappear later. It is also possible that if the stress (the source of the problem) is left untreated, it could manifest itself in some other form of suffering, such as headache, anxiety, short temper, mental distraction, etc.

Patanjali also recognized that we need more than one tool to address suffering effectively, because every person is different. What may be appropriate for one person, need not be useful for another.

For example, a physically healthy person would be able to do some postures, no doubt. But *asana* is less useful for a person with limited mobility, as in the case of Steve after his stroke. But there were other tools available for Steve. Just because he could not do *asana*, did not mean he could not do yoga.

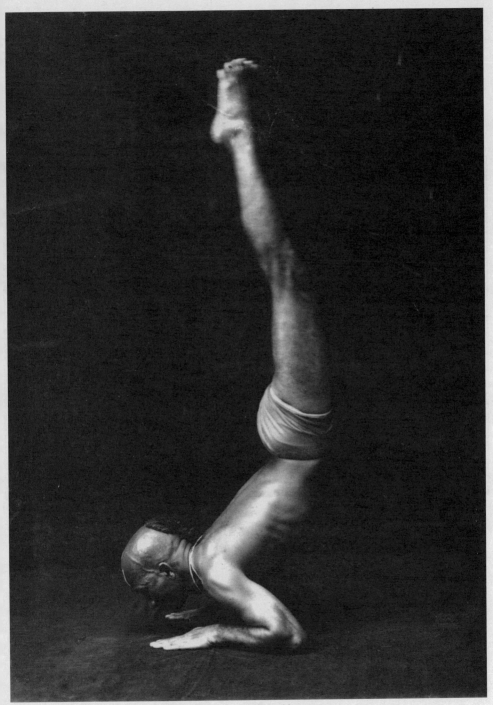

Krishnamacharya, also a master of *asanas*, demonstrating *Pinca Mayurasana*.

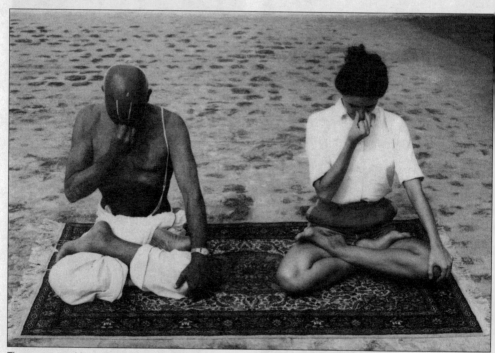
The master teaching *pranayama* to a female student.

This is why Patanjali offers a wide range of tools for use in yoga. I will present a few of them here, briefly.

dhyanam: meditation

According to Patanjali, meditation is the most important tool in yoga. Of the 195 aphorisms in the *Yoga Sutra*, only three are about *asana*, seven discuss *pranayama*, and the rest of the text is devoted to meditation. Patanjali elaborates on the different types of meditation, the qualities of a focus, the benefits of the various focuses, etc.

A brief definition of meditation might be: an intensive process that involves choosing a focus and linking with it on a deep level. Meditation does not happen automatically. *Asana* and *pranayama* are considered good preparation for meditation.

asana: postures

Asana is one of the most popular tools of yoga today. *Asanas* are careful arrangements of the various parts of the physical body, and so *asana* is primarily a practice for the physical body. *Asana* postures can be done dynamically or statically, and each posture has its own benefits. There are an infinite number of postures, but only a few hundred of them are practiced regularly today.

In *asana* practice, the postures are supposed to be done with careful regulation of breath, allowing the student to experience the full benefits of the pose. So, although *asana* is primarily a physical practice, it influences more than our physical body.

pranayama: conscious regulation of breath

We are breathing all the time, but we are not doing *pranayama* all the time. *Pranayama* is the practice of consciously regulating the different components of the breath—inhalation, exhalation, and retention of breath—for a specific duration of time, so that the resulting breath is long and smooth.

For example, we may exhale twice the duration of inhalation, or we may want to do equal duration of inhale and exhale, then hold after exhale. *Pranayama* is one of the most powerful tools of yoga.

yama: social attitudes

Cultivating good habits in our social lives is very much a part of yoga. In many situations, our suffering is the result of poorly-made choices in our social relationships. This is why the five *yama* were offered, so that we may practice them in our life and avoid suffering. Non-violence, honest communication, not stealing, being faithful to a partner in a relationship, and non-coveting make up the five aspects of *yama*.

niyama: personal attitudes

Another source of suffering is our attitude towards our self. We are tormented by low self-esteem, lack of confidence, etc. These emotions dramatically impact our daily lives. The five *niyama* are suggestions for nurturing healthy personal attitudes. These include cleanliness of body and mind, contentment, a clear lifestyle that keeps the body free of toxins, self-inquiry, and refined action.

pratyahara: sensory control

Pratyahara is appropriate usage of the senses. For example, if we abuse our senses or if we do not use them at all, we get into trouble. A friend of mine lost much of his hearing ability, because he would listen to music in his room with the volume turned all the way up for hours and hours at a time.

Through certain practices like *pratyahara*, we are taught to regulate the senses in such a way that they function appropriately and serve our needs. Rather than controlling us, we control the senses.

ahara niyama: dietary recommendations

A big part of how we feel or what we feel depends on the food we eat. Are we eating the right food, at the right time? Are we eating too little or too much? These are all questions that need to be addressed if we want to live a healthy life. This is why the role of *ahara niyama* is so important.

vihara niyama: lifestyle recommendations

Just like food, lifestyle is an important factor in our well-being. What kind of job do we have? Are we getting enough rest? Do we get to spend time with the family? Do we have a hobby that we can pursue? Our problems often stem from poor lifestyle choices, and if we make better choices, our problems disappear.

bhavana: visualization

Visualization is often used as part the process of healing or directing the mind. *Bhavana* are very powerful, because the mind is a more powerful tool than the body. For instance, when a student whose hands were paralyzed came to us, she was given a practice that included visualization. We asked her to visualize her hands moving up during inhalation and visualize them lowering during exhalation. Such use of visualizations helped her begin to move her arms again after a few months.

mantra japa: recitation of special sounds/hymns

Sound produces vibrations in the body, and these vibrations stimulate different areas of our human system. This is especially true with Sanskrit sounds, which are phonetically-based, rather than alphabet-based. Correct pronunciation is crucial, because these sounds, correctly pronounced, produce specific vibrations that act on specific areas of our system. These sounds need not be religious in nature. They may be simple syllables or other sounds that have a meaning for us. For example, we could use a sound that honors a force in nature, like the sun.

mudra: use of gestures

There are many gestures used in yoga. Some of them are called *bandhas*, which are often used in *pranayama*. Others involve placing of the hands or the feet in special positions that have a symbolic

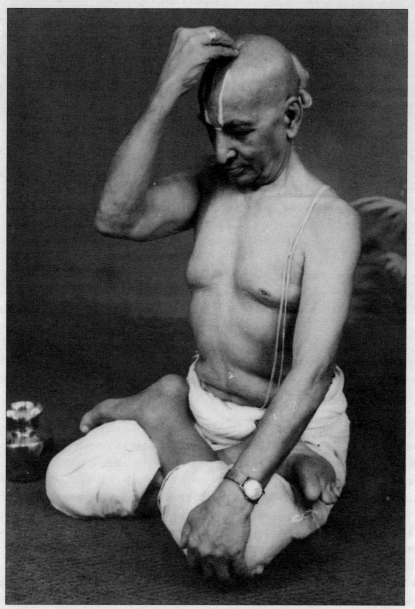
Krishnamacharya demonstrating the use of symbolic gestures in practice.

meaning. These are extremely useful for working with people with certain problems, such as Parkinson's disease. A person with Parkinson's disease experiences a great deal of trembling in the body, especially the arms. When we use certain *mudras* and ask them to retain the gesture for some time, their whole attention focuses on doing that simple movement. They consciously hold the hand in that gesture, when usually the hand would be trembling unconsciously. In this way, the *mudra* slowly helps them to better control their condition.

Many of these gestures also have a hidden meaning, which we may discover through constant practice of such gesture or by meditating on them.

svadhyaya: self-inquiry through counseling

This is a very important tool in yoga. We often get into trouble because we fall into certain patterns of behavior that we are not conscious of. We don't see our behaviors, because they are so much a part of us and have become habitual. This is when the help of a trusted, competent counselor becomes very important. Through *svadhyaya*, we may discover what our problems are, and then we can solve them by making changes in our life.

yajna: ritual

In some cases, we get into trouble because there is no order in our life. Life is full of chaos and everything is in disarray. This is when ritual comes to our aid. When I speak of ritual, I do not mean religious rituals, although they may be a part of practice for those who believe in God. Ritual means simply to become more aware of our daily actions and to perform them mindfully.

For example, before we eat, we can take a moment to thank Mother Nature for being so generous. This makes us more mindful of our eating, and also creates a good attitude in us before we eat. This enhances the quality of our digestion and our health.

These are some of the most common tools in yoga mentioned in the *Yoga Sutra*. I have not listed all of them, nor have I gone into great detail with the ones I have covered, as this falls out of the scope of this book. However, it is important for us to recognize that there are many tools in yoga. In order to be a truly competent yoga teacher, you need to understand most of them and become skillful in using them. Once we do this, the possibilities are endless, and we can begin to see the amazing potential of yoga.

Steve's story is an example of yoga's potential to heal. Steve was unable to make many physical movements or perform postures, but he could do breathing practices or *pranayama*, and so this is where his teacher began. She taught him simple breathing exercises that he could practice while lying in his bed. Masters of yoga believed that breathing practices affect the state of mind profoundly, and as Steve diligently continued with his simple *pranayama* practice, his mind began to be affected in a positive manner.

Once Steve was comfortable with the breathing techniques, his teacher introduced some visualization or *bhavana*. She asked him to visualize that while he was breathing in, the breath would move to the left side of his body. While he was breathing out, she asked him to visualize the breath moving from the left side of the body, outward.

This is just one of the many examples of *bhavana* that Barbara practiced with Steve over a period of time, and they dramatically influenced Steve's condition. He reported feeling the effect of these *bhavana* practices for the first time during one of his acupuncture sessions. He had never felt the needles before, but soon after beginning the visualizations, he started to feel them. Not long after that, he was making minor movements with his left hand and leg. This was amazing, not just to him, but also to the healers working with him.

In yoga, there is a belief that mind is more powerful than matter. Here, the visualization that Steve was doing during his breathing engaged his mind and helped direct his attention to the area of his body that needed healing, and it began to heal. This is an example of how the body functions holistically.

I discussed this story with one of our neurosurgeon friends, Dr. B Ramamurthy, who recently passed away. I asked him if this could happen, and he answered emphatically, "Yes it is possible." He went on to explain that when the mind becomes engaged in this kind of a visualization process, the brain sends out healing signals to the body, and this is how the healing occurs. He said that scientists are now trying to learn more about this process.

By this time, I had met with Steve and started working with him in collaboration with Barbara. Once he began to move his limbs a bit, we introduced simple movements. Again, we coordinated the physical practice with breathing, as well as with visualization.

Steve's stubbornness came in handy. As he put it, "Some days, I would feel very heavy and my body would not want to do some things. But my mind would not give up, and I wanted to do the practice. Only after the practice, I would realize how good it was that I was stubborn. The practice would make me feel lighter, even in the body."

One day, Steve told me something that resonated with what the *Yoga Sutra* has to say about how yoga heals holistically. When I asked him if he enjoyed his yoga, he said, "I look forward to my yoga sessions the most. For me, I feel that yoga takes away the role of many of the other healers working on me. The movements I do in yoga replace the job of the physiotherapist working on me. When I do some sounds with the movements that Barbara asked me to do, I realize that I don't need a speech therapist any more. When I do my *pranayama* and visualizations in the practice, I feel so calm that the psychologist does not have to come and calm me down any more. **Yoga seems to be an all-in-one package.**"

This is one of the biggest advantages of yoga. It is a holistic system that addresses multiple dimensions of the body at the same time. When you are raising your hands coordinated with breathing and using visualization in the mind, you are not just working on the physical body, you are also influencing the breath

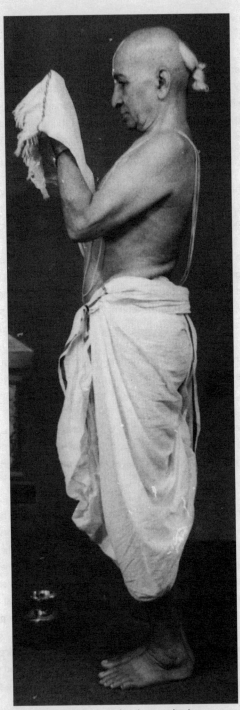
Krishnamacharya practicing the sun ritual.

and involving the mind in the healing process. The practice becomes more powerful, more potent; it is not a mere physical workout.

This is why Steve began to heal so much more quickly when he took up yoga, because yoga addresses multiple needs at the same time. The other healing techniques required that he spend hour after hour with different specialists, working on one problem at a time. This approach to treatment often left him tired and frustrated.

After two years, during which I carefully monitored his progress, Steve returned to his job. He had improved so much that the company felt he was fit enough to return to work full-time. He rediscovered his passion for fly-fishing and hiking. He gave up his partying days, though. He told me that he only parties with his "yoga friends, as the drinking is minimal or nonexistent."

While the classical yoga masters understood the powerful healing potential of yoga, by the early twentieth century, many people thought yoga was just a bunch of physical postures, and nothing more. Convincing people that yoga was much more than that was not going to be an easy task. The young Krishnamacharya would need a lot of support and blessings from a higher force if he were going to revive interest in the ancient yoga tradition. Fortunately, these would come in the form of his teacher at the summit of the world.

The Himalayas.

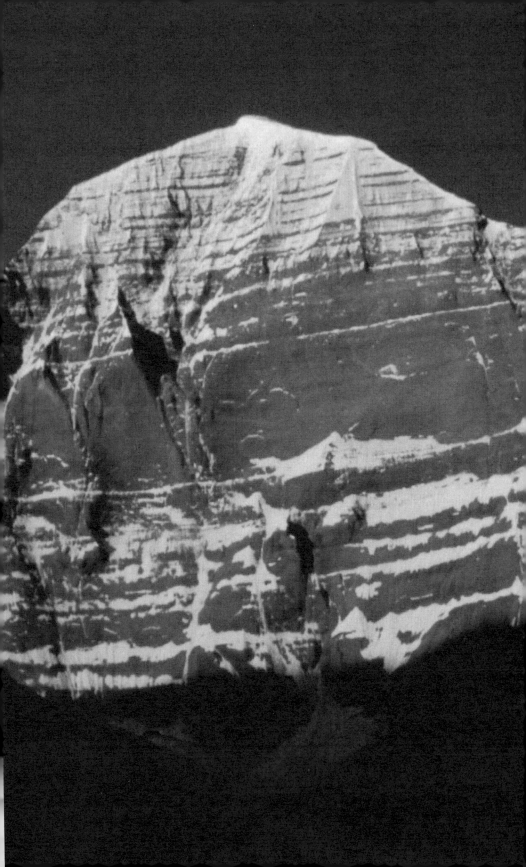

Chapter Three

Northward Bound
maturing into the yoga master

mountains are where the truth is.

The incident at Alvar Tirunagari changed Krishnamacharya's life forever. It was clearer than ever to him that he was destined to play a role in resurrecting the glorious tradition of yoga just as his ancestor Nathamuni had revived *Sri Vaisnava Sampradayam* centuries before. But this was not going to be an easy task for a sixteen-year-old young man, and Krishnamacharya realized that if he was going to be successful, he had to continue learning in order to build up his knowledge and credentials.

He returned to Mysore, resumed his education and quickly mastered many subjects. He took examinations to complete various *sastras* (traditional subjects) at the *Vidvan* (Professor) level, which in those times was an extraordinary achievement. Even at this highest level, however, he was not satisfied. The well of India's ancient teachings ran deep, and he recognized that all of these teachings, including yoga, were connected to each other. If he did not master the entire spectrum of India's philosophical teachings, it would be difficult to fulfill his goal. It was at this point that Krishnamacharya resolved to be a full-time student and cast away all other ambitions.

It was usual in those days for a person to take a job as a professor once he passed examination at the *Vidvan* level, but Krishnamacharya was not interested. His interest was wisdom alone, and he was a man in a hurry to acquire that wisdom. Logic (*Tarka*), Grammar (*Vyakarana*), and *Samkhya* were some of the subjects he wanted to pursue more intensely. Studying the *Yoga Sutra* thoroughly was another top priority, and he had strong memories of his father's discourses on yoga from this sacred text.

Krishnamacharya continued serving at the Parakala Math while pursuing his *Vedanta* studies in greater depth under Pontiff Vagisa Brahmatantra. But before long, he expressed a desire to move on to Varanasi (also called Benares) and pursue his studies there under the city's famed scholars. Varanasi was considered one of the most holy places in the country, and also a seat of great learning. Almost every great scholar or academician would go there to study and learn.

The Pontiff gave Krishnamacharya permission to go, and in 1906, he was bound to Varanasi. At Varanasi, he learned Sanskrit Grammar (*Vyakarana*) from Siva Kumara Sastri, a great master of the language and an ardent devotee of Lord *Narasimha* (another incarnation of Lord *Visnu*).

There is an interesting story connected to this period of Krishnamacharya's life. Siva Kumara Sastri called Krishnamacharya to him one evening and taught him all of the rare and secret aspects of the Sanskrit language in that one, single night. Strangely, the very next day, the master lost his speech forever. It appears that he had been waiting for a deserving student to whom he could transfer these secret teachings, and once he had done that, his voice left him as if it were of no use anymore. After this experience, Krishnamacharya pursued his study of Logic (*Tarka*) with a master called Trilinga Rama Sastri, before returning to Mysore in 1909.

In Mysore, Krishnamacharya continued to delve deeply into the ocean of knowledge. He pursued his studies of *Vedanta* with the new Pontiff, Sri Krsna Brahmatantra, with whom he would also take long walks around Mysore. Under the Pontiff, Krishnamacharya studied the *Upanisads*, the *Bhagavad Gita*, and other very important *Sri Vaisnava* texts, including the *Rahasya Traya Sara*, composed by Vedanta Desikacarya.

At the same time, Krishnamacharya was enrolled in Mysore University studying various subjects. From Mysore, he earned the title *Veda Kesari* (one of the highest titles given to someone who is well-versed in the *Vedas*) and the title *Mimamsa Vidvan* (Scholar of *Mimamsa*, one of the six schools of Indian philosophy).

In 1914, Krishnamacharya's pursuit of knowledge took him back to Varanasi. He was now a handsome young man of twenty-six years.

The never-ending quest for wisdom is epitomized by *antevasin*, one of the Sanskrit words used to describe a student. Translated literally it means, "one who stays until the end." This definition can be interpreted in many ways. Most often it is interpreted as "one who stays with the teacher until the end of education." It can also mean, "one who stays with the teaching until the end." This is the meaning of *antevasin* that best describes Krishnamacharya.

In Varanasi, Krishnamacharya lived in Radha Krishna Mandir Assighat and continued his education at Queen's College. Every day he woke up early in the morning to walk the six miles to the college. He attended classes from 6:00 a.m. until 10:00 a.m., and then walked back home.

It was tradition in those days for students to beg for their food, and this is how Krishnamacharya and the other students fed themselves each day. They lived far from home with no steady income, so society at that time determined that it was a good idea for them to beg for food from different houses. The families in the area would not hesitate to perform this service, because at one time, they probably had done the same. Also, they knew that their own children would be students in need of this service in the future.

This system had many advantages. First, it helped the students focus on their education, instead of worrying about procuring food. Also, visiting with so many families helped the students learn that each house was different, the people inside were different, the way they lived was different, the way they communicated was different, etc. It was an excellent lesson in sociology.

Finally, the requirement to beg ensured that the students remained humble by forcing them to depend on the kindness of others for their survival. Begging also taught them generosity, and after they completed their education and began to raise a family, they would find themselves on the other side, providing meals for begging students. They would remember the generosity of those who had fed them and be generous in turn. Students no longer beg for their meals today, but the practice served its purpose.

Krishnamacharya's teachers at Queen's College were Sri Vamacarana Bhattacarya and the principal of the college, Sri Ganganath Jha. Ganganath Jha suggested to Krishnamacharya that he apply for a scholarship reserved for the most outstanding students. The scholarship examination was given in Hindi language, but Krishnamacharya requested special permission to take the examination in his native tongue, Telugu. The college granted his request, and among the sixty-three people who took this test, only three of them passed. One of those three was Krishnamacharya. The scholarship provided him the peace of mind to pursue his education with even greater fervor.

The following year, Krishnamacharya passed the examination to qualify as an *Upadhyaya* (Teacher). Armed with this success and the credentials he'd already earned, he took the post of assistant lecturer, and Ganganath Jha requested that he teach his own son, Amarnath Jha.

Dedicated as he was to pursuing his education, Krishnamacharya also took time to enjoy life. Every summer, he traveled to the Himalayas and visited temples and other holy places. He loved to walk and enjoy the beauties of nature. Over the course of his long life, he would travel far and wide, visiting every corner of India. He believed that travel was one of the best teachers a person could have, and he always encouraged his own students to travel.

While Krishnamacharya was teaching and studying in Varanasi, his father's discourses and the memories of his classes on yoga were often on Krishnamacharya's mind. He still practiced the *asanas* and *pranayama* his father had taught him.

One day, a local saint who had noticed Krishnamacharya practicing yoga, directed him to a renowned *yogi* named Sri Baba Bhagvan Das. Krishnamacharya met with the *yogi* and expressed his desire to learn and take the highest examinations in Yoga. Impressed by Krishnamacharya's eagerness and qualifications, Sri Baba Bhagvan Das allowed Krishnamacharya to present himself as a private candidate and take the examination in *Samkhya* and Yoga at Patna University.

Krishnamacharya passed the examination with distinction. His teachers at Varanasi, Vamacarana Bhattacarya and Ganganath Jha, were amazed at his ability to absorb so much knowledge in such a short time.

But Krishnamacharya's thirst for yoga was not quenched. He sought the help of Ganganath Jha, who was not only the college's principal, but also a *yogacarya* (yoga master). Krishnamacharya told Ganganath Jha that he wanted to follow his father's advice and master the *Yoga Sutra*.

Ganganath Jha advised him, "If you really want to master yoga, you must travel beyond Nepal to Tibet. This is where a *yogi* called Rama Mohana Brahmacari lives. He is the only one who can teach you the complete meaning of the *Yoga Sutra*."

Krishnamacharya wanted to leave immediately, but it was not easy in those days to travel out of India. He had to wait a little longer and hope for some luck.

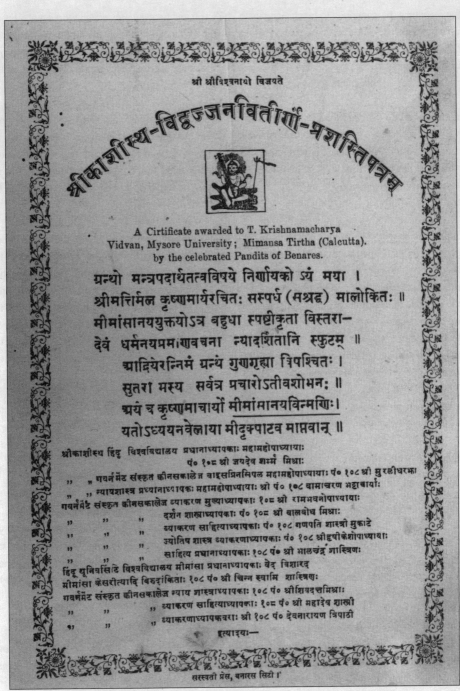

श्री श्रीविश्वनाथो विजयते

श्रीकाशीस्थ-विद्वज्जनवितीर्णा-प्रशस्तिपत्रम्

A Cirtificate awarded to T. Krishnamacharya
Vidvan, Mysore University ; Mimansa Tirtha (Calcutta).
by the celebrated Pandits of Benares.

ग्रन्थो मन्त्रपदार्थतत्त्वविषये निर्णायको ज्यं मया ।
श्रीमन्निर्मल कृष्णमार्यैरचितः सस्पर्धं (सश्रद्धं) मालोकितः ॥
मीमांसानययुक्तयोऽत्र बहुधा स्पष्टीकृता विस्तरा—
देवं धर्मनयप्रमाणवचना न्यादर्शितानि स्फुटम् ॥

च्याद्रियेरन्निमं ग्रन्थं गुणगृह्या त्रिपश्चितः ।
सुतरा मस्य सर्वत्र प्रचारोऽतीवशोभनः ॥
अयं च कृष्णमाचार्यो मीमांसानयविन्मणिः ।
यतोऽध्ययनवेळाया मीदृक्पाटव माप्तवान् ॥

श्रीकाशीस्थ हिंदू विश्वविद्यालय प्रधानाध्यापकाः महामहोपाध्यायाः
पं० १०८ श्री जयदेव शर्मे मिश्राः
" " गायर्नमेंट संस्कृत कीनसकालेज वाइसप्रिन्सिपल महामहोपाध्यायाः पं० १०८ श्री मुरलीधरका
" " न्यायशास्त्र प्रधानाध्यापकः महामहोपाध्यायाः श्री पं० १०८ वामाचरण भट्टाचार्यो
" गवर्नमेंट संस्कृत कीनसकालेज व्याकरण मुख्याध्यापकाः १०८ श्री रामचन्द्रोपाध्यायाः
" " " दर्शन शास्त्राध्यापका पं० १०८ श्री बालबोध मिश्राः
" " " व्याकरण साहित्याध्यापकाः पं० १०८ गणपति शास्त्री मुकाटे
" " " ज्योतिष शास्त्र व्याकरणाध्यापका पं० १०८ श्रीहृषीकेशोपाध्यायाः
" " " साहित्य प्रधानाध्यापकाः १०८ पं० श्री भालचंद्र शास्त्रिणः
" हिंदू यूनिवर्सिटि विश्वविद्यालय मीमांसा प्रधानाध्यापकाः वेद विशारद
मीमांसा केसरीत्यादि बिरुदांकिता १०८ पं० श्री चिन्न स्वामि शास्त्रिणः
" गवर्नमेंट संस्कृत कीनसकालेज न्याय शास्त्राध्यापकाः १०८ पं० श्रीशिवदत्तमिश्राः
" " " व्याकरण साहित्याध्यापकाः १०८ पं० श्री महादेव शास्त्री
" " " व्याकरणाध्यापकवरा श्री १०८ पं० देवनारायण त्रिपाठी
इत्यादयः—

सरस्वती प्रेस, बनारस सिटी ।

One of the certificates awarded to Krishnamacharya by the "celebrated Pandits of Benares."

In the meantime, he continued to teach Ganganath Jha's son and nephew, while also working at a library for one hour each day. This library work had been arranged through an important gentleman, Kumbakonam Sri Rajagopalacarya, who was very close to the King of the state. Hearing of Krishnamacharya's accomplishments and dedication, the King offered him a state job, but Krishnamacharya respectfully declined. He had set his sights on going to Tibet to meet his teacher.

Krishnamacharya's desire to travel to Tibet was growing so strong that he finally requested permission to leave. He approached a gentleman called Srinivasa Iyengar, manager of the East India Railway Company, and requested a railway pass. So impressed was the gentleman with Krishnamacharya's qualifications and his deep desire to travel to Tibet, he issued a letter that enabled Krishnamacharya to use the railways to travel anytime, anywhere. He felt that this was the least he could do to help this young man on his quest.

With permission from his teacher and other associates from the college and a railway pass in his hands, Krishnamacharya headed north to the Himalayas. He traveled via Simla, the summer headquarters of the British Viceroy, in order to acquire the papers he would need to leave India. Ganganath Jha had given him a letter addressed to the Viceroy introducing his young student as a candidate known for his proficiency and knowledge of the different Indian schools. In the letter, Jha requested the Viceroy's help obtaining the travel documents that would allow Krishnamacharya to travel on to Tibet. Unfortunately, the Viceroy was sick with diabetes, and Krishnamacharya was forced to wait until he recovered. The doctor handling the case was Devedra Bhattacarya, the son of Vamacarana Bhattacarya, one of Krishnamacharya's teachers at Varanasi. So, a ray of hope remained.

One day, Krishnamacharya received an invitation from the Viceroy. Hopeful, he arrived at the appointed hour, and right away, the Viceroy asked him, "How much yoga do you know?"

Without a moment's hesitation and with great pride, Krishnamacharya answered, "I may not know as much as India needs, but I know enough to teach foreigners."

Impressed with the young man's confident answer, the Viceroy began taking yoga classes with him. In about six months time, his diabetes was under control. The Viceroy was so happy with Krishnamacharya, that he made arrangements for him to cross the Himalayas and proceed to Tibet, taking care of the expenses himself. The Viceroy also sent two aides to escort Krishnamacharya on his arduous journey. Before Krishnamacharya departed, the Viceroy asked him to return once every three months, so that he could continue his studies with the skillful young teacher.

In all of the documents that are either part of Krishnamacharya's own handwritten archives or part of the oral records taken down as notes by some of his students, the name of the Viceroy has never been mentioned. This is probably due to the fact that convention in India dictates that we must never address the King or the ruler by their actual name. Since the Viceroy was the de facto ruler of the country, ruling on behalf of the British Empire, no one, including Krishnamacharya, would have addressed him by name, only by title. However, in my research, I found that this particular Viceroy must have been either Lord Hardinge (Viceroy from 1910 to 1916), or Lord Chelmsford (Viceroy from 1916 to 1921).

On his way to Tibet, Krishnamacharya visited the Muktinarayana shrine and bathed at the origin of the river, Gandaki. Here, he found a *Saligrama*.

Saligrama stones are fossil stones characterized by the presence of discus marks inside them. They are worshipped in temples, monasteries, and households all over the world as visible and natural emblems of *Visnu*. They are also used in quasi-religious functions like house-warmings, marriages, and funerary rituals. They are found only in the river Gandaki, a Himalayan stream. It is believed that a person who offers a daily service for the *Saligrama* stone will be freed from the fear of death, and he will cross over the stream of births and deaths. Finding such a holy stone on his way to meet his teacher was indeed an auspicious omen for the young Krishnamacharya.

From here, Krishnamacharya continued on his way, and after twenty-two days and a trek of 211 miles, he finally reached Manasarovar. It was here that he would find his teacher.

I have often wondered how Krishnamacharya made this journey. Even today, with so much sophisticated equipment available to hikers, a journey like the one he undertook is considered difficult and exhausting.

On a recent trip to Mysore, I met up with one of Krishnamacharya's students, Pattabhi Jois, to interview him for this book. When I brought the conversation around to the subject of Krishnamacharya's visit to Mt. Kailash, he burst into tears and said, "No one will be able to do that journey today. Krishnamacharya made this journey in times when you did not have proper shoes, when you did not have packed food available. Only his determination to find his *guru* took him there. Such faith is rare today."

Even after his long and tiring journey, Krishnamacharya did not rest when he reached Manasarovar, but set out to find his teacher's dwelling. Eventually, he came across a cave and standing at the entrance was a very tall hermit with a long beard. The hermit wore wooden shoes and was looking out with a face of great calmness. Krishnamacharya knew immediately that this was his teacher.

Krishnamacharya prostrated before the hermit and requested to be accepted as his student. The man questioned Krishnamacharya in Hindi, asking him why he had come all the way to Tibet.

When Krishnamacharya recounted his story and his deep desire to learn everything there was to learn about yoga, the hermit called him into the cave. Inside, he met his teacher's wife and three children. They welcomed Krishnamacharya and his aides with fruits called *ankula* and served them tea. Afterwards, the escorts set off on their return journey.

The long-awaited moment had arrived for Krishnamacharya. He had finally found his teacher, and his joy knew no bounds. The master took Krishnamacharya to the famed Manasarovar Lake and showed him around the places nearby. Krishnamacharya was surprised that he still had not experienced cold or fatigue from his journey. "Perhaps it was due to the intake of the fruit or the grace of my *guru*," he would later recount about this experience.

Krishnamacharya's first instruction from his teacher was to take a bath and perform *acamana* before the first precept of *pranayama* could be taught.

Acamana is a simple daily ritual performed by many Indians. It includes taking three sips of water and touching different parts of the body while reciting various *mantras* (chants). Though there are many religio-spiritual reasons behind this practice, it also has practical applications, one of the simplest being to wet the throat before *pranayama*. If the throat is dry, the practitioner may start coughing. Also, by touching different parts of the body, we bring our attention to them and notice if they are in order.

For eight days, the master would teach Krishnamacharya nothing but *pranayama*. He also instructed Krishnamacharya to eat only fruits. Krishnamacharya accepted his *guru's* direction without hesitation.

Later, he would understand that his *guru* had instructed him in this manner in order to teach him patience, a very important virtue to cultivate in the process of learning and practicing yoga. In traditional teaching systems, the teacher would always test the student before accepting him or her in order to make sure that the student possessed the faith and commitment necessary to pursue education with the teacher. If there were no faith and no commitment, it would be a waste of time for both teacher and student to continue any further.

After those eight days, Krishnamacharya was accepted and became a part of his teacher's family. His daily food from that point on consisted of *chapatti* (Indian bread) and *halva* (a paste of vegetables or fruits sweetened with ghee and sugar or honey).

Some people might think the *guru's* test pointless. Krishnamacharya had already proven his commitment by making this difficult journey. When I asked my father about this, he said, "Firstly, you don't question the teacher's testing methods. Secondly, maybe the teacher was testing if Krishnamacharya had come to him with a desire to learn that was ego-based, rather than a desire to learn with the intention to use that wisdom to serve society."

I asked my father, "Do you think for Krishnamacharya it was based on ego?"

"If so, he would not have been accepted by his teacher," my father replied swiftly.

Krishnamacharya's period of study with his teacher lasted seven and a half years. Rama Mohana Brahmacari made him memorize the entire *Yoga Sutra*, *Yoga Kuranta* (a text in Nepali language), and other

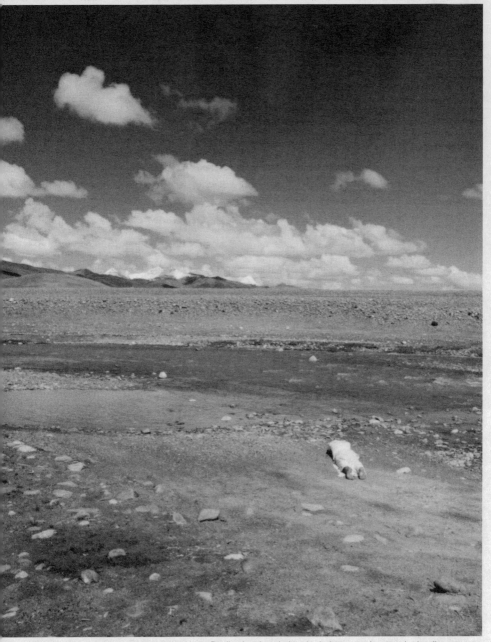
is custom that one prostrate to Mt. Kailash. Here, Desikachar is saluting the holy mountain, seen in the distance.

important yoga texts. According to Krishnamacharya, *Yoga Kuranta* contained a wealth of information, including how to adapt *asana* and *pranayama* to suit the different needs of individuals, and how to use certain aids (props in today's parlance) to help in the healing process. Krishnamacharya wrote this himself about this now lost text, and his words contradict the popularly held notion that the *Yoga Kuranta* was the basis for *Astanga Vinyasa Yoga*.

Krishnamacharya did not forget his promise to the Viceroy to return to Simla once every three months. His *guru* gave him permission to make this journey, and even sent his son, Ramacandra Bramhacarya, to accompany Krishnamacharya on these trips.

Only when Krishnamacharya had learned all the texts by heart did Rama Mohana Brahmacari teach him the deeper meanings of each one. At the same time, Krishnamacharya was also learning the advanced yoga practices, along with many tools of yoga (not just *asana* and *pranayama*), such as *cikitsa krama* (therapeutic tool). This was a period in his life and education when Krishnamacharya began to mature into the yoga master he would become.

This must have been an incredible experience for Krishnamacharya. The Himalayas are very lonely and peaceful. Only the most daring are interested in traveling there, and those who do only attempt the journey in the summer months when roads are still accessible and the weather bearable. It has not changed much since Krishnamacharya visited there, except maybe it was a little lonelier then, than it is today.

I often wonder how Krishnamacharya survived in such a place for so long. "It was the grace of my *guru*," he recalled later. "It was his blessings, the practice that he taught me, and the care with which I was taken care of by his family that helped me during these years. I am forever grateful to them for this."

I also think about how intense this period of study must have been for Krishnamacharya. Imagine living with your teacher and his family for over seven years. There were no printed books, no notebooks or computers to learn from or take notes in. You learned everything from your *guru*, and you memorized what he taught you. As you are doing all of this, you are also being watched, observed, evaluated, and corrected by this perfectionist master. If you needed a break, there were no distractions like television, radio, bars, restaurants, etc. To get away, you hiked up one of the giant mountains that were also the backdrop for your everyday life and practice. It was a very congenial arrangement for studying yoga, a subject that requires a lot of disciplined practice, meditation, and self-inquiry, but it is a situation very few would want to be in today, even if it were possible.

After spending nearly eight years of his life learning from and serving his teacher, Krishnamacharya was summoned by his master.

"I am happy with your educational progress," Rama Mohana Brahmacari told him. "Now go back to society, lead the life of a married man and spread the message of yoga. This is the *Guru Daksina* I want for what I have taught you."

Guru Daksina, or payment to the teacher, was a very important aspect of education. In those days, when the teacher demanded the *daksina*, that signalled that the student's education was over. Often, what was demanded from the student depended on the student's resources. Payment was not always in cash. It could be a cow, or a house, or some other form. In some cases, as in the case of Krishnamacharya, it might even be a task. The teacher never asked for more than the student was capable of giving, and the student never departed without paying or fulfilling the *daksina*. It was considered blasphemous if the student did not pay his due.

Heeding his teacher's words, Krishnamacharya returned to India in late 1922. The only souvenirs he brought back from his long stay in Tibet were the teachings he learned from the master, his memories, a pair of wooden sandals belonging to his teacher, and a set of drawings of various *asana* poses drawn by his teacher's daughter.

The wooden sandals of the teacher represent the teachings of the teacher himself. They serve as a reminder of the teacher, as well as of the humility the student must show before the teacher and the teaching. Krishnamacharya never forgot this. Every day of his life from that point on, he woke up, completed his morning rituals, and before beginning his work, he would humbly place the sandals of his master on his head. This was an act of humility, but for Krishnamacharya it was also a way of cherishing the precious moments with his master.

Krishnamacharya knew that it was time to return home and share what he had learned from his teacher. He also knew that an extraordinary task still lay before him. To be a yoga teacher for life would be a great challenge and convincing people that yoga was not just a set of postures, but something with much more depth and potential, was going to be even more difficult. Although his yoga education was complete, he needed to build his credibility as a master and this required further study. He decided to return to Varanasi and continue his education before committing to yoga full-time. He was determined to take up different degrees from the Universities of Calcutta, Allahabad, Patna, and Baroda.

In Varanasi, Krishnamacharya was welcomed with great warmth by Ganganath Jha, Vamacarana Bhattacarya, his teachers, as well as Gopinath Kaviraj, the University Vice-Chancellor. He quickly turned his attention to his goal and spent those first six months back in India in Calcutta. The principal of the college there, Sri Naliniranjan Chatterji, was initially skeptical of Krishnamacharya, but he was cordial to him, since he had been highly recommended.

Before long, Chatterji was so impressed with the new student that he sent his own daughter and three other students to study yoga with him and arranged for a scholarship.

Two former colleagues at the college, Laksmana Shastri and Ananthakrishna Shastri, however, were opposed to Krishnamacharya taking the examination without fulfilling the four-year attendance requirement. But Sri Chandrachud Tarka Tertha, the Professor of Logic, spoke in Krishnamacharya's favor, arguing that

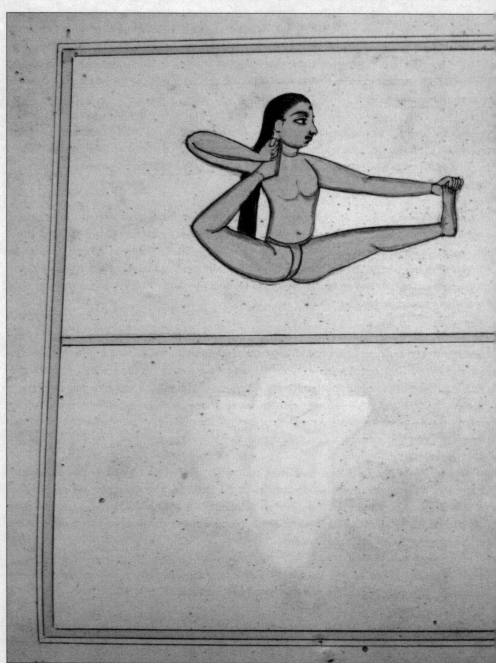

A souvenir from Krishnamacharya's trip to Mt. Kailash, the book of drawings made by his teacher's daughter.

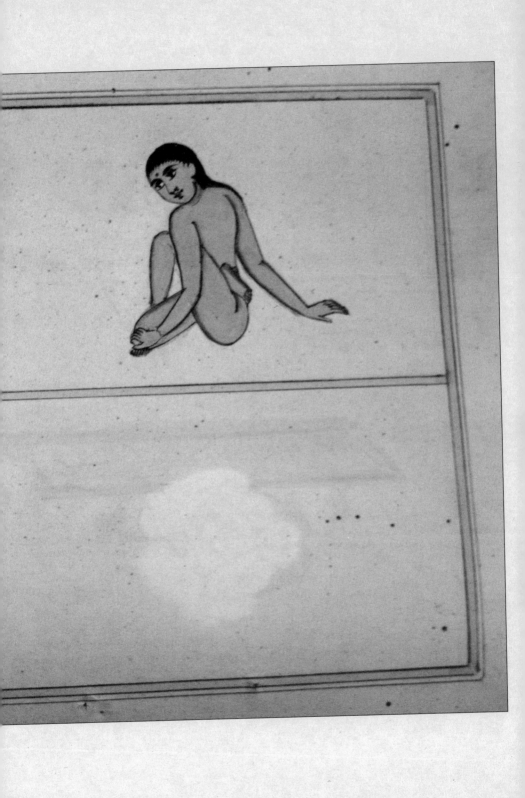

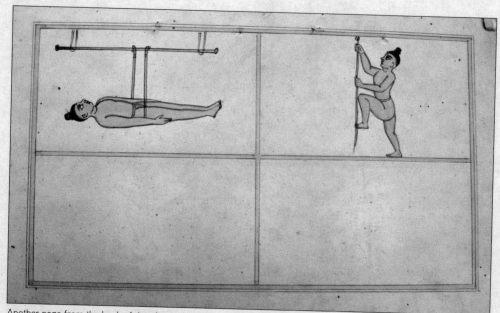

Another page from the book of drawings, showing that the use of props, like ropes, was prevalent even in those days.

he had the capacity to do the four-year course within a year. Krishnamacharya did not let him down. He completed the *Mimamsa Tirtha* examination in only nine months, in February 1923.

During the final oral examination, Ananthakrishna Shastri abruptly ended the exam after hearing Krishnamacharya expound majestically on the *Sabara Bhasya* (an important commentary on *Mimamsa*). Right there, he announced that Krishnamacharya had passed. The four-day oral examination was completed in a single day. Krishnamacharya was unable to attend the convocation, however, as he was scheduled to take the examination for the *Nyayacarya* degree (Professor of the School of Logic) at Allahabad.

Krishnamacharya's reputation was spreading fast. Many acknowledged his prowess as a scholar and an authority on the different *sastras*. His skills were called upon many times by people who wanted him to settle disputes based on various teachings. One such dispute concerned the kingdom of Vijayanagar.

The *Maharaja* of Vijayanagar, Sri Alaknarayana Gajapathi Singh of Andhra, had passed away suddenly. Family tradition required following the instructions of the *Bodhayana Sutra*. According to this teaching, every *krama* needed to be preceded or accompanied by *Kusmanda Homa* (a very special ritual). However, the officiating priest, Rayudu Subha Sastri, said the ritual need not be performed in this case, and that it was sufficient if the *mantras* alone were recited. The *Maharani*, not satisfied with the decision, referred the matter to the Hindu Dharma Samsthapana Committee of Benares.

Sri Gurulinga Shastri, the president of the committee, was studying *Mimamsa* under Krishnamacharya. He approached Krishnamacharya, who agreed to resolve the dispute after first obtaining permission from his teacher, Sri Vamacarana Bhattacarya. Having done so, he had to justify his conclusions to three experts, Muralidhara Jha, Kasi Prabhudatta Agnihotri, and Ganesh Maratha. They suggested that he write a treatise on "What is *Mantra*?" Meanwhile, Muralidhara Jha, the Vice-Chancellor, had also asked six other teachers to write on "*Bodhayana Sampradaya*" and "*Mimamsa Sampradaya*."

The teachers were given eighteen days to write their treatises. On the nineteenth day, the treatises were presented before all of the *Mahamahopadhyayas* (teachers of the teachers). The first meeting was at Kamakotipitha, Hanuman Ghat in Varanasi. Three South Indian and three North Indian scholars presented their papers. The results were announced in the presence of thirty-two *Mahamahopadhyayas* from Calcutta, Benares, Madras, Mysore, and Baroda. Sri Ganganath Jha presided and announced the results.

"Our student from South India, Krishnamacharya, has written a treatise called *Mantra Padartha Tattva Nirnaya*, and this has been adjudged the best presentation." The titles *Mimamsa Ratna* (Jewel of Mimamsa) and *Nyayacarya* (Professor of Nyaya) were immediately conferred upon Krishnamacharya, and he was presented with a gold medal and a certificate from the Government College. The treatise he wrote helped resolve the dispute between the *Maharani* of Vijayanagar and the officiating priest.

Krishnamacharya would soon have to settle another dispute, this one more personal. After the examination, Krishnamacharya met his uncle at Varanasi. His uncle brought the message that the Pontiff of the Parakala

Math, Vagisa Brahmatantra, had passed away and that Krishnamacharya was asked to take over as the next Pontiff.

This was a tricky situation. Usually, when you are asked to be the Pontiff, especially if you come from a long line of revered spiritual masters, you cannot refuse that position. It would be very inappropriate. However, Krishnamacharya's teacher had asked him to raise a family and teach yoga. If he became Pontiff, he could not have a family, because this position required him to remain single. Also, if he became the Pontiff, he would not be able to dedicate his life to yoga. Instead, he would have to dedicate his life only to the *Sri Vaisnava* tradition.

Once again, Krishnamacharya needed a miracle, and the miracle came in the form of an ancient Indian quotation that he remembered.

> **siveruste gurustrata, guroriste na kascana**
>
> *if you let down the Gods, the teacher will still be able protect you,*
> *if you let down the teacher, no one will be able to save you.*

Taking solace from this message, Krishnamacharya refused the exalted position and continued on his journey.

In 1924, Krishnamacharya traveled to Baroda for his *Veda Kesari* examination. At that time, there was a famous university at Navadvipa in the state of West Bengal staffed by learned scholars. Krishnamacharya wanted to go there for a degree in *Nyaya Ratna* (Jewel of Nyaya).

Instead of spending an entire year at Navadvipa, his teacher's son, Devandra Bhattacarya, advised him to study in Benares and go to Navadvipa only for the examination.

Krishnamacharya completed his degree successfully and was granted the title *Nyaya Ratna*. His teacher was Vagisa Bhattacarya, who was the *guru* of Vamacarana Bhattacarya.

After bathing in the confluence of the Ganga and the Bay of Bengal, Krishnamacharya moved on to Haridwar. From Haridwar, he went to Gangotri and Yamunotri, and then proceeded to Tibet to see Rama Mohana Brahmacari, who permitted him to return to his own country for good.

On his return, Krishnamacharya was introduced to the *Maharaja* of Patiala, who took him to the Amristar Mandir, the most sacred place of the Sikhs and explained the history to him.

In that same year, Krishnamacharya went to see the *Maharaja* of Dholpur on an invitation from the King himself and taught him yoga for a month.

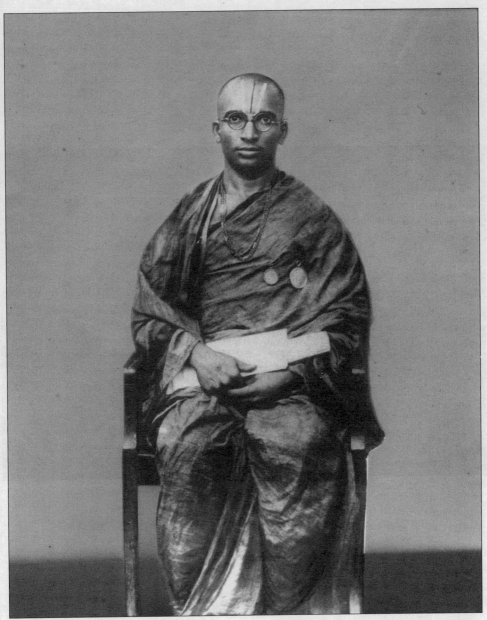

Krishnamacharya with all of his certificates and medals, just before his marriage.

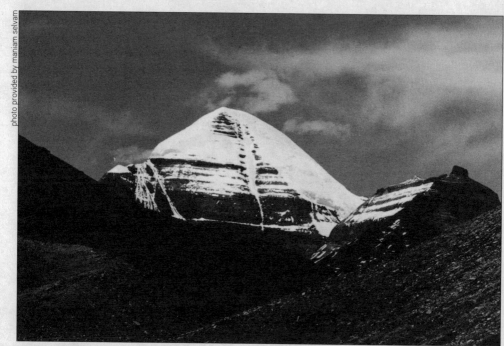

Another view of Mt. Kailash, where Krishnamacharya spent nearly eight years.

After Krishnamacharya's return to Benares, the *Maharaja* of Jaipur, hearing of his reputation as an outstanding scholar and yoga expert, called him to serve as the Principal of the *Vidyasala* (School of Education) in Jaipur. This arrangement, with its regular schedule of classes and the necessity of answering to many different people, did not suit the free-spirited Krishnamacharya. The anniversary of his father's death was approaching, and he decided to return to Varanasi to perform the necessary rituals at the Ganga.

Krishnamacharya was courted by various Kings impressed by his skills and knowledge and was frequently honored by his community. In August 1924, *Mahamahopadhyaya* Sri Gurulinga Shastri arranged a debate on the *Mata Traya* (three philosophies), *Murti Traya* (three idols), and *Sthana Traya* (three places). Krishnamacharya argued against Sri Rudhra Bhatta, a passionate debater. After hearing the arguments from both sides, the judges declared Krishnamacharya the victor. They presented certificates to him and praised him as the only student to have obtained such a wealth of knowledge since the founding of the college.

It was at this moment that Krishnamacharya decided his formal education was complete. He had not only completed a long period of study with his yoga master, he had earned the highest degrees in all of the Indian philosophical schools. He was also proficient in *Ayurveda*, Astrology, music, many languages, and other ancillary teachings.

It was time to leave Varanasi and return to Mysore for good. Mysore was the city in which he had grown up, and it would also be the city where his fortunes would change forever.

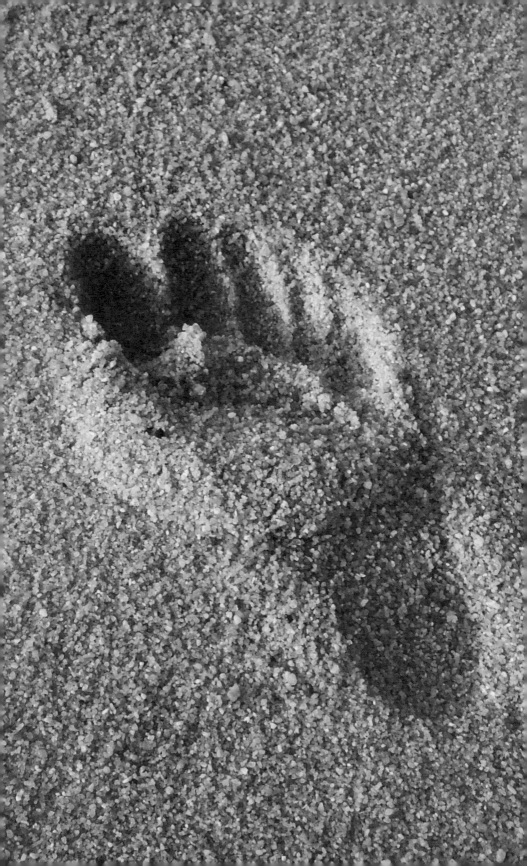

Chapter Four

One Size Does Not Fit All
finding the yoga that's the right fit

we are each a unique social being.

"It does not work," rebuked the man in the neck brace.

I was shopping in a mall and was surprised to be addressed in such an aggressive way by someone I had never seen before in my life.

"Excuse me," I said to him, "are you talking to me?"

The man nodded. "Yoga does not work. Look," he pointed at his neck. "Look at what it has done to me."

It took me a moment to figure out why this man was talking to me in the first place, then I realized I was wearing a T-shirt that made the bold statement **"yoga works."**

My curiosity was piqued. I asked the gentlemen to explain why he had made such a strong statement about yoga. He invited me to sit down with him and told me his story.

"I have had this neck pain for the last three years of my life. I have tried many things to make it better, but it just won't go away. One of my friends at the office suggested I try yoga. She said that her neck was bothering her a few months ago, and that she took some yoga classes and her pain vanished. She assured me that my neck pain would go away, too, if I did yoga. I knew my gym was offering some kind of yoga classes to their members, so I enrolled. We did one-and-a-half hours of various postures, and the very next day, my neck was in such bad shape that I had to get this collar. This is why I say 'yoga does not work.' And, by the way, I'm Peter."

I introduced myself as a yoga teacher, and then I asked Peter, "Did you tell the teacher that you had a neck pain?"

"No," he replied.

"Did you check to see if this class was an appropriate one for you?"

Peter looked at me as though I was crazy and said, "Aren't they all the same?"

I shook my head. "Peter," I said to him, "we need to have a talk."

There are many people like Peter. They think that walking into any yoga class will work for them, but this is not the case. If we walk into a doctor's clinic, and he offers us the same pill he gives to everyone else, would we accept it? And if we did accept it, would it be appropriate for us?

No way.

Yoga is not a "one-size-fits-all" practice. As I pointed out in a previous chapter, yoga views the human being as more than just the physical body. The human system is multidimensional. There is not only the physical body, but a breathing body, the personality, an intellectual dimension, and an emotional dimension, and all of these dimensions are interconnected. For this reason, it is not always the case that when pain is expressed in one dimension, the root of the problem must also be located in that same dimension.

For example, in the case of Peter, I found out that the source of his problem was not his neck, but his highly stressful job and lifestyle. The pain in the neck was only a manifestation of the stress that he was dealing with in his life.

However, in the case of his friend, it turned out that she had a spasm in her neck, because she had exposed her neck to cold wind for too long. So, though the pain is similar, we see that the cause of her problem is quite different from the cause of Peter's. This is why a yoga practice that worked for her did not work for Peter. All Peter's friend needed was some warm circulation in her neck, and probably, the postures she did in her yoga class facilitated this. That's why she would have agreed with my T-shirt, "yoga works."

Also, we need to keep in mind the fact that Peter's friend was a lithe and lightweight woman in her early thirties. Peter, on the other hand, was tall, stiff, and definitely not very light. So when he went to this yoga class, he practiced some postures that were inappropriate for him and aggravated his existing neck problem.

This is why, traditionally, yoga was offered on an individualized basis. The ancient masters focused on the question of how to apply yoga, because the approach to each student would be different depending on the intention of the practice. Even when working with a group, even with a shared intention, the abilities and needs of each individual student in the group were respected. If the masters had not committed themselves to teaching in this manner, if the ancient texts had not emphasized the appropriate use of yoga, Peter would be right and **yoga would not work.**

Yoga is a powerful tool, and the more powerful a tool is, the more potent it can be, or the more dangerous. It depends on the way we use it. Consider a very sharp knife, for example. The sharper the knife is, the more delicately it can cut, if used appropriately. Or, the more easily it can hurt someone, if used carelessly. We cannot blame the knife for being too sharp. We just need to make sure we use it appropriately.

The same principle holds true for yoga. Yoga is a powerful, helpful tool. Use it appropriately, and it works wonders. Use it carelessly and inappropriately, and you can hurt yourself and others.

Below are the six categories into which the ancient masters divided yoga, based on the focus of the practice. These are basic categories, with no discussion of the tools that might be used within in each category, because the combinations are endless. Any combination would be based on the needs and abilities of the individual student and so would differ in each case.

srsti krama

In *srsti krama*, the focus is on growth: physical, mental, psychological, and emotional. Often *srsti krama* is introduced to children. The intention is to gain strength and flexibility, sharpen the mind and make it more attentive, and strengthen and begin to learn subtle control of the breath. A person given *srsti srama* as their practice would be very young and healthy.

siksana krama

Here, the focus is perfection—be it postures, *pranayama*, *bandhas*, or any other tool of yoga. The goal is for the practitioner to use the tools of yoga without error. Often, teachers introduce *siksana krama* to young, healthy adults. One of the main reasons this practice is introduced to students of a young age is so that they will learn to practice yoga and use its tools correctly. Then, they are taught how to modify these tools. This is a very useful practice for teachers.

raksana krama

Raksana means maintenance or sustenance. The focus of *raksana krama* is maintenance of health, relief of stress, and rejuvenation. This practice is ideal for most adults with families and busy social and professional lives. At this stage of life, our primary need is to maintain our health, so that we can fulfill our responsibilities.

adhyatmika krama

Here, we practice yoga to discover and nourish our spiritual side. There comes a point for many of us when we start to wonder about spiritual issues. We are looking for something deeper in life, and we want to connect with it. It is at this moment that we embrace *adhyatmika krama*, which focuses on helping us move forward on this spiritual journey.

cikitsa krama

Cikitsa means "therapy," and *cikitsa krama* focuses on the use of yoga in the healing process. If we are working within this category, then we are experiencing problems with our physical, mental, emotional, or psychological health. We have some kind of unease/disease that we want to get rid of. The focus here is returning to a state of ease and health. Steve's story is a classic example of *cikitsa krama* used appropriately and successfully.

sakti krama

Only a few, elite yoga masters have practiced this category of yoga, and the only *yogi* I have ever met who did was Krishnamacharya. In *sakti krama*, yoga is utilized to develop and enhance certain "*sakti*" or "*siddhi*" (special powers). When my father, Desikachar, asked his father, Krishnamacharya, to teach him some of the *siddhis* like stopping the heartbeat, my grandfather replied, "This is not so useful for society now. I will only teach you what is useful." Though he did not teach *sakti krama* to my father, Krishnamacharya demonstrated on more than one occasion that *sakti krama* is indeed possible.

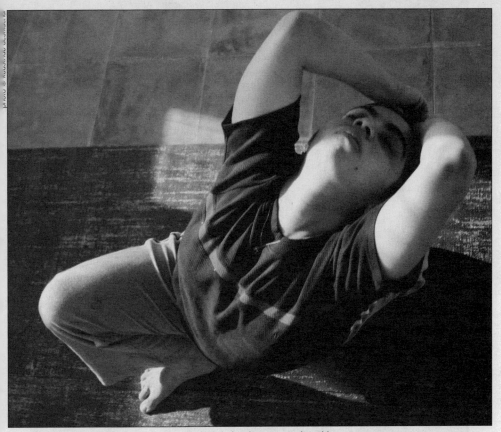

Mekhala Desikachar performing an intense back arch that forms part of *srsti krama*.

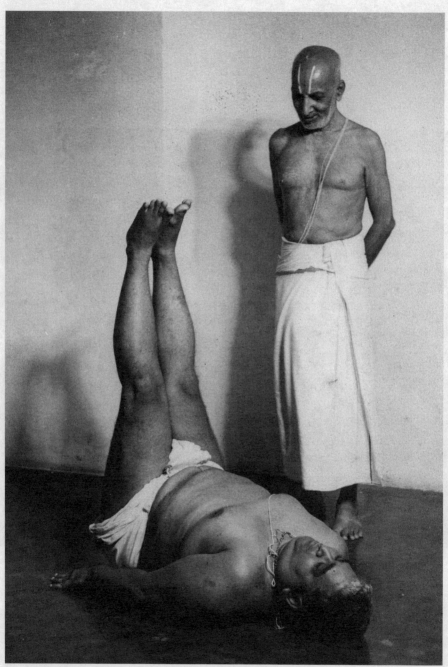

Krishnamacharya teaching yoga as a *cikitsa* (therapy) to one of his students.

If we look at the map of our own lives, keeping in mind the six categories of yoga practice, we clearly see that *srsti krama* may be most appropriate when we are very young. *Siksana krama* would become our focus when we are in our late teens or early adulthood. *Raksana krama* may become more relevant for our adult life, and as we age, we may find ourselves drawn more to *adhyatmika krama*. Whenever we need some therapeutic help, we can call on *cikitsa krama* to set us right.

Of course, these categories are only guidelines. There are always exceptions. A person can be interested in *adhyatmika krama* even when very young or pursue *srsti krama* and *siksana krama* in adulthood.

Also, there will always be occasions when there is overlap between the categories, and there is not a clear line of distinction between one level and another. For example, if I have a job and I need that job to sustain my family, there is no way I can stop working. But if I contract an illness, then I will become very tired while I am working, so I may have to do elements of *raksana krama* to rejuvenate myself each day, while still focusing on *cikitsa krama* so that I can heal from my illness as soon as possible.

I asked my father about his own personal practice, and how it had changed over the years. He was very generous not only in sharing his experience with me, but also in allowing it to be shared with others through this book. He said, "I will be happy to share this information, but I have one suggestion for the reader. Just because I went through this evolution in my own practice, it does not mean that everyone will go through the same process. They must find their own practice and its evolution through the guidance of their own teacher."

"Another important issue here is that my studies with my teacher were never only practices. So many aspects were attended to, right from the beginning—memorizing of yoga texts, learning them with their meaning, how to practice different components of yoga, and how to apply them, etc. But since you ask me about my personal practice and its evolution, I will stick to that domain."

After a brief pause, my father continued. "I began to be interested in yoga early in the 1960s, when I was in my early twenties. I was very thin and quite fit. In the early days of my yoga practice, my father taught me what is known as *siksana krama*. I had to do all the postures and *pranayama* perfectly. No mistakes were allowed. If I could not do some posture correctly, I would be prepared for it using other postures so that it would become perfect. He never pushed me into doing [a posture] correctly through force. It was all very gentle, but perfection was definitely the goal. Since I was very fit and flexible, within a few years, I was able to do most of the *asanas* and *pranayama* correctly. This included doing them with the *bandhas*, and with specific ratios of breathing so that I would master them totally."

"By the early '70s, my practice had shifted completely from *siksana krama* into what is called *raksana krama*. This is probably because my father began to notice that I was getting a bit older (now in my early thirties), and also that my work load had increased—I was already a full-time yoga teacher with quite a few students. Another important factor was that I was now married, and I already had my first son. So,

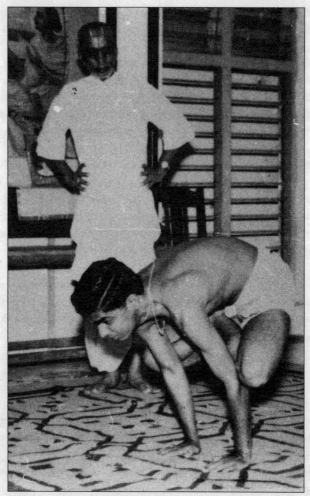

Desikachar performing *siksana krama* under the eagle eyes of his father.

here the practice was mainly focused on *pranayama*, but also included a reasonable amount of *asana* practice and also a brief component for silent meditation. Looking back, I think this was invaluable to me because this is exactly what I needed. I would have gone crazy if not for this kind of a practice. My life was already becoming more and more busy and just to keep up with it, as well as with the arrival of two other children within the next ten years, meant that I needed some magic to keep me going. This is what came in the form of my practice. My father would constantly monitor my practice and change it time and again to suit my current needs. However, beginning in the early '70s until the mid '80s or so, the practice I have been doing is totally in the realm of *raksana krama*."

"By the late '80s, I had already changed quite a bit in my approach to life and outlook. In my earlier days, I had shunned anything religious or spiritual. But after so many years of practicing yoga in such a profound manner, as well as dealing with people from all walks of life practicing all kinds of belief systems, the spiritual side which was hiding within me began to show itself. I think my father noticed this, and one day, he called me and taught me a practice which was in line with the principle of *adhyatmika krama*. It consisted of a very special practice that included a bit of *asana* and *pranayama*, but heavily loaded with meditative components like *japam* (repetition of *mantra*), *dhyanam* (meditation), and *yajna* (ritual). I have been doing this practice since that day, and I think I am beginning to understand its profound effect on me."

"The beauty of *adhyatmika krama* is that it takes time to show results in you. We can see quick results in the other two *kramas*, but in *adhyatmika krama*, it is not so quick. We need patience, perseverance, and dedication to practice it regularly. Though I began this late in the '80s, I began to see the effects of it only later in the '90s. These changes are very personal, and hence, I would prefer not to share it. It will also sound like arrogance if I started talking about it, and hence, I would prefer my actions to speak about these changes, rather than my words."

I was quite moved by this exchange, and I can assure readers that having lived with my father since I was born, I know that he has changed a great deal, especially since the late '80s. He developed an uncanny intuition—he always seems to be right. His patience with people has greatly increased, and his perception is extremely refined, especially the ability to see subtle changes in people and in society at large. So, I know that deep changes have taken place in him, probably due to his inwardly-focused practice.

At another sitting, I asked my father if he had ever pursued *sakti krama* and *cikitsa krama*. My father laughed and answered, "I tried to get my father to teach me *sakti krama*, especially how to stop the heartbeat. He refused to teach saying that this was not useful for the benefit of society. He asked me to focus on and learn about *cikitsa krama* instead, which will be of great service to society. So I learned a lot about *cikitsa* from him over the years. I have also benefited from *cikitsa krama* time and again. Since I started traveling, there have been days when I have ended up with some kind of sickness—either a back pain, or a cough, or extreme fatigue. In such cases, I have definitely relied on *cikitsa krama* to get relieved of such sickness. However, I have learned a lot about *cikitsa krama* from my father and have seen

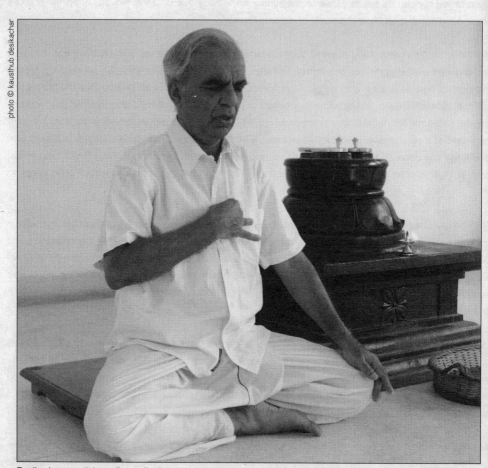

Desikachar practicing *adhyatmika krama,* which includes meditation, chanting, and the use of gestures.

its powerful benefits by sharing it with people who have had much worse health problems. People have avoided surgeries, come out of severe migraines that have bothered them all their life, have worked out of severe depression, battled cancer using yoga as a great support system, and even become calmer despite being HIV positive. *Cikitsa krama* has been an integral part of my learning and evolution since the 1960s, as I have been dealing with sick people from the very beginning of my journey in yoga."

What these stories make clear is that in order to be a yoga teacher, we need to spend a reasonable amount of time learning from a competent teacher who can teach us what is most appropriate for us.

This is why Krishnamacharya went to such extremes to educate himself; he wanted to be a good teacher. A teacher needs patience and must spend a reasonable amount of time being a student before he/she can become a good teacher. A teacher should also be able to judge what kind of yoga her student needs, and teach him accordingly.

Many people ask me if two hundred hours is enough training for a yoga teacher. As a reply, I usually pose this question: "Would you go to a medical doctor who has trained for only two hundred hours?"

Most of the time, the answer is, "No way."

There is never enough training. We must constantly learn and intern with our teacher, so that we become better teachers with each passing day. This is why even modern medicine has continuing education. Continuing education is vital if you want to be a good healer in any healing discipline.

When I raised this issue of "When is one ready to be a yoga teacher?" to my father, he replied, "I began to teach when my teacher asked me to teach. I knew that I knew very little yoga to teach, but I had the backing of my teacher who would guide me in the process. We cannot actually learn swimming until we enter the swimming pool. Nor can we automatically start swimming once we are in the pool. However, the swimming coach will not put us into the pool, if we are not ready to enter it. Similarly, when we begin to learn yoga, the teacher will consider our strengths and weakness and provide us the opportunity to teach at the right time. Once this happens we must not lose contact with the teacher. We must continue to be monitored and learn from the teacher for as long as possible. I began my teaching in the 1960s and continued to learn from my father until he died in 1989. If he were alive today, I would still be studying with him. This is because yoga is a vast ocean. It is not a simple set of tools that can be easily learned and repeated. **We need continuing education.**"

When I asked him about people who did not have such easy access to the teachers, my father told me, "The thirsty man will definitely find his water. Similarly, the one who is really eager will definitely find the right teacher and learn from him. Even Krishnamacharya traveled many miles to find his teacher. I agree that, in today's context, we can't leave our families for years to study with our master. We need to find a balance. My suggestion would be to find the right teacher, spend a reasonable time with him/her in the

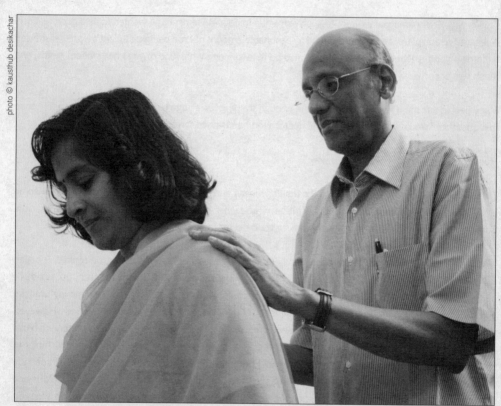

S Sridharan, Managing Trustee of KYM, testing a student before *cikitsa krama* (Yoga Therapy) is performed.

beginning, and then keep in constant touch by returning regularly. This way, your education will evolve, be up-to-date, and you will be doing the best service to your own students."

In the Krishnamacharya Yoga Mandiram, the center founded by Desikachar in honor of his father, the teacher-training program lasts two years. However, the most important aspect of this program is that each trainee has a mentor with whom they pursue their private practice, seek answers and clarifications, and grow as a teacher. These mentors themselves have mentors, and hence, the chain is continuous. It is this system of continuing education that makes teachers here very special. I am sure that this model can be replicated all over the world.

It is easy to be a simple yoga instructor these days, but being a complete yoga teacher is something different. Krishnamacharya showed us through his life's work how vast yoga's potential is, and when applied appropriately, how powerfully it works in every aspect of our being. Thanks to his efforts, it is easier for us to become better yoga teachers. All we need is the thirst and the patience.

When I explained the different categories of yoga to Peter, he was amazed.

"I did not know we had so many choices in yoga. I guess I just went into a class that was not appropriate for me," he said.

His voice was friendlier now, and he asked me to get a cup of coffee with him. As we walked to Starbucks, I asked him, "Would you come here if all they sold was one kind of coffee in one size?"

Peter smiled and ordered, "One grande-skim-mocha, no whipped cream, light on the chocolate."

I was glad he got the message.

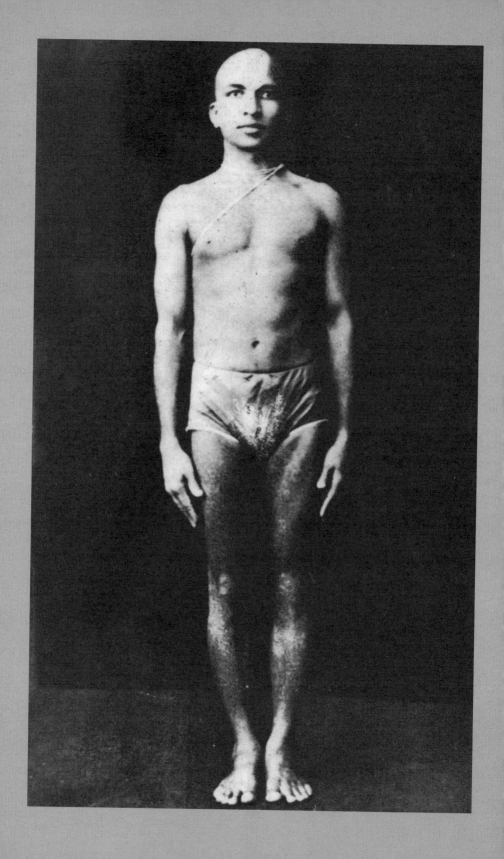

Chapter Five

A Regal Beginning
laying the foundations for the
golden era

get it right the first time,
for life may not give you a second chance.

Equipped with degrees from the best universities in India, Krishnamacharya was ready to commit himself to fulfilling his teacher's command. He wanted to dedicate his life to yoga.

But at a time when few were interested in yoga, would he find anyone in Mysore to whom he could teach what he had learned? Krishnamacharya did not worry about this question, because he believed strongly that if he followed his teacher's direction, everything would happen as it should.

The *Maharaja* (King) of Mysore, Sri Krishnaraja Wodeyar, had come to Varanasi to celebrate his 60th birthday, accompanied by his mother and an entourage of relatives, courtiers, ministers, and other aristocrats. The King had heard of Krishnamacharya's accomplishments and knew of his eagerness to return to Mysore, so he invited him to come to the palace. Krishnamacharya accepted the invitation, and soon, he became the yoga teacher for the *Maharaja* and his family. Krishnamacharya's teacher had indeed blessed him with a good benefactor.

When Krishnamacharya told his family and friends in Mysore that he was dedicating his life to yoga, they were shocked. Some even told him he was crazy. He heard the same comment over and over: "With your qualifications in the *sastras* you can become head of any educational institution or even a minister in the court. Why are you wasting time being a yoga teacher?"

Krishnamacharya's family and friends were so concerned about his choice, because yoga was not popular in those days. It paid very little and was not considered a respectable vocation. However, to Krishnamacharya all of this was immaterial. To become a yoga teacher and to raise a family was the only *Guru Daksina* his teacher had asked of him in return for his education. There was nothing else he wanted to do. So, in 1925, he fulfilled his teacher's second request and married Namagiriamma, a young girl nearly twenty-five years his junior.

Child marriage was very common in India in those days. Although girls were married off at a very young age, real family life began for the married couple only after the young woman was grown and ready to take on such responsibility. This type of arrangement between a girl and an older man was considered practical for both parties. The father was typically quite old by the time his children reached adolescence, and because it was believed that a daughter needed to be protected, the family wanted to secure her future early on. This way, if her father died, a husband was already in place to take care of her.

It was different for sons. At the time, Indian society believed that boys could be on their own and take care of themselves. A young man went out into the world and sought a teacher and an education until he was nearly twenty-five or thirty, so that he was able to offer himself as a worthy husband and provider. In the case of Krishnamacharya, when he returned to Mysore he was nearly thirty-seven, and he more than matched the qualifications that Namagiriamma's parents were looking for in a prospective husband for their daughter.

While teaching yoga in Mysore, Krishnamacharya was offered the position of Pontiff of the Parakala Math twice more. He politely refused both offers. For someone born into a lineage long committed to serving in the *Sri Vaisnava Sampradayam* tradition, it was unheard of to refuse such an offer. This offer was considered not just an honor, but a duty. Krishnamacharya's decision confused many of the people around him, but he was not discouraged. He knew that his teacher's blessings would protect him, even though the path ahead was not going to be easy.

He may have refused the call to serve as Pontiff three times, but Krishnamacharya did not give up *Sri Vaisnava Sampradayam* as part of his personal religious practice and studies. He found many of the teachings of the *Alvars* to be consistent with the teachings of yoga that he had received from his master in the Himalayas. Over time, he integrated the message of the *Alvars* with the message of yoga.

For example, when teaching the *Yoga Sutra*, he would talk about dedication to God as one of the paths Patanjali offers for reaching the state of yoga. For those who believe in God, he would tell his students, this is the easiest path. If we devote ourselves to God completely, in the sense of *prapatti* or "total surrender" (as mentioned in the *Sri Vaisnava Sampradayam*), the need for other yoga tools in our practice will be minimal.

However, Krishnamacharya knew that this path would not appeal to everyone. Only those who believed in God would be willing to attempt it. So, he did not insist that his students follow this path, but he did offer it as an option to those who were drawn to it. In this way, he showed respect for yoga, which requires the teacher to honor the beliefs and path of each student.

In the meantime, he continued working for the *Maharaja*. He proved himself an extremely competent healer and counselor, and soon became one of the *Maharaja's* most trusted advisers. It was with the *Maharaja's* encouragement and help that Krishnamacharya established the *Yoga Shala* (School of Yoga) in the Mysore palace.

The *Yoga Shala's* purpose was to promote yoga and its benefits to the public. There were classes for young boys and girls, as well as adults, and classes for the healthy, as well as for those who sought Krishnamacharya's therapeutic counsel. He instructed the young boys and girls separately in a large hall and held private consultations in a smaller room nearby. He also trained some of his students to become instructors, especially in *asana* and *pranayama*.

Krishnamacharya taught many things to his students at the *Yoga Shala*, and what he chose to teach depended on the focus of the group or the individual he was working with at the time, in accordance with the teachings of Nathamuni and Patanjali. To the group of youngsters who came to him in the mornings and evenings, he taught dynamic postures linked together in smooth, organic sequences. The students were required to master all of these sequences. Two of these students from Krishnamacharya's *Yoga Shala* are regarded today as great *yogis* in their own right: **Pattabhi Jois and BKS Iyengar.**

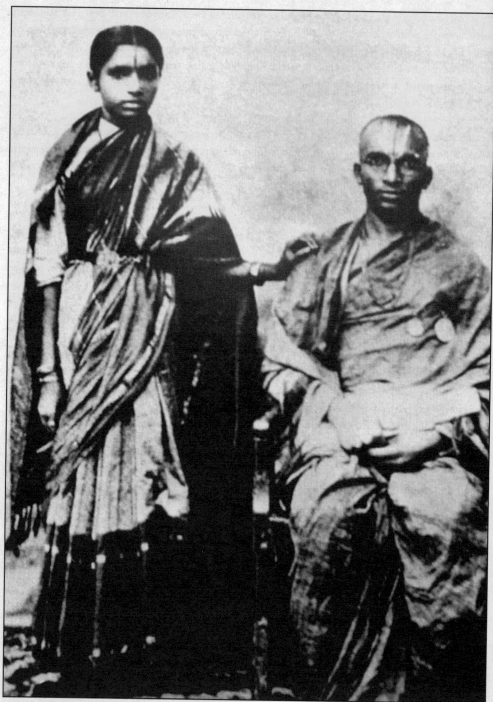
Krishnamacharya and Namagiriamma after their wedding.

Krishnamacharya's young students often demonstrated their progress for the King, who eventually asked Krishnamacharya to record the postures he had taught his young students in a book. This is how Krishnamacharya came to write his first book, *Yoga Makaranda*, (*Honey of Yoga*) in 1934. *Yoga Makaranda* details the *asana* sequences that he taught these young boys and girls in the *Yoga Shala* in the 1930s. Many of these sequences are practiced today as "*Astanga Vinyasa Yoga*," but they originated in Krishnamacharya's *Yoga Shala*.

Krishnamacharya also traveled all over the state of Mysore during this time, lecturing on various topics related to yoga as part of his efforts to reintroduce yoga to his fellow Indians. During each lecture, students like BKS Iyengar and Pattabhi Jois would help him demonstrate various postures and sequences. Later, his own children, Desikachar, Sribhasyam, and Sri Shubha, would accompany him when he lectured and demonstrate poses for the audiences.

From conversations I have had with BKS Iyengar and Pattabhi Jois and from reading anecdotes provided by his students and friends, it is clear that Krishnamacharya was a strict and demanding teacher. One incident that Iyengar related to me illustrates this.

"In one of the demonstrations," Iyengar told me, "we were two students who had to perform postures. I was good in some of them, while Keshava Murthy was good in many of them. He was one of Krishnamacharya's pet students. However, he ran away the day before this demonstration, and the entire responsibility fell on my shoulders. *Guruji* [Krishnamacharya] gave me the list of postures that we would do the next day. However, [before] the actual demonstration happened, he completely changed the list. I was flabbergasted, but could not open my mouth. I somehow managed everything, except the last one, *Hanumanasana*, which was difficult for me because my shorts were quite tight. When I told him about this he just took me to the side and ripped my pants in the sides so that [they] would loosen a bit. Then he said, 'Now you can do it.' Such was the intensity of my teacher, Krishnamacharya."

I was surprised at this story. I had always known my grandfather as a very sweet man. Since I was his grandson, maybe he did not show this side to me, or maybe he had changed with age. On a recent visit to Pune during BKS Iyengar's 85th birthday celebrations, I asked him again about Krishnamacharya's disciplined approach, wanting to know if it had affected him positively or negatively.

"Had it not been for the intensity of my *Guruji*," Iyengar replied, his voice strong and clear, "I would not be what I am today. It was the intensity that he passed on to me that has helped me progress in the yoga path. I owe it to him. Even though it was painful in those days to receive it, I am reaping its benefits now."

Pattabhi Jois offered me a similar view of Krishnamacharya. When I met him in 2003 while traveling with some of my students, one of them asked him if Krishnamacharya had been strict with him.

"Very strict," was his prompt answer. After a moment's pause, he continued, "But only for the sake of

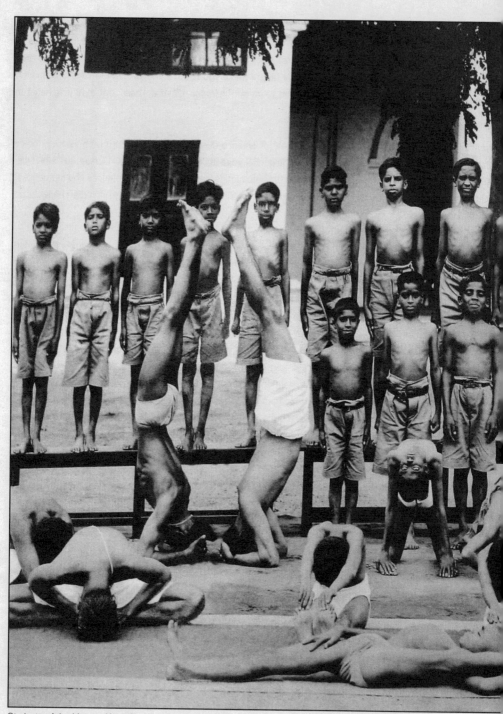

Students of the Mysore *Yoga Shala* performing various *asanas*.

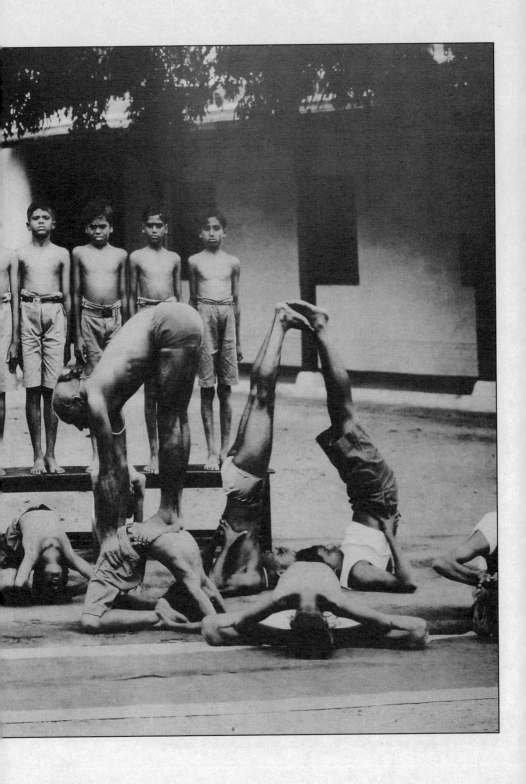

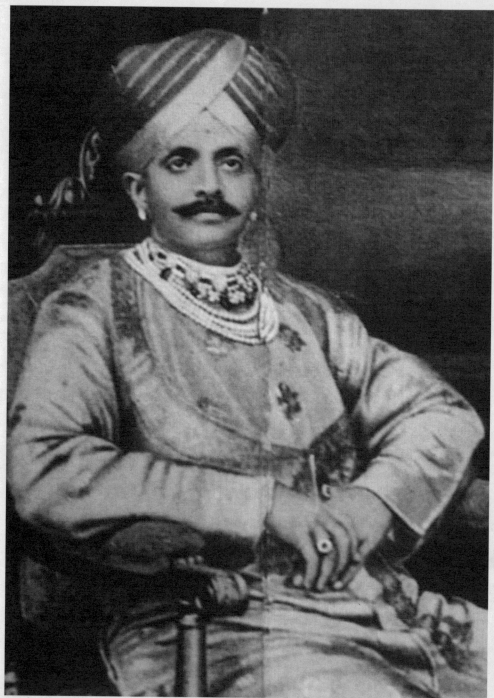
Krishnaraja Wodeyar, the *Maharaja* of Mysore, a patron and student of Krishnamacharya.

dharma (duty). He wanted us to be the best. This is why he was strict. He would make us do the *vinyasas* perfectly. If we made mistakes, he would ask us to repeat it again, until it was right. But outside the classroom, he was a very kind man. He would give us food and teach us *sastras*."

Krishnamacharya may have been strict with his students, but this strictness, his emphasis on discipline, and his intensity were all born of love for the teachings. His teacher had expected the very best from him, and so he demanded the same from his young students and teachers, inspiring them to become teachers of the highest calibre.

Krishnamacharya did not teach the same things to the healthy adults and the Royal Family at the *Yoga Shala* that he taught to his young students and trainee teachers. When working with the healthy adults, he focused more on *raksana krama*, teaching some simple *asanas*, but mainly *pranayama*, and also some meditative practices. He would design individualized practices combining these elements for each student.

In addition, each student performed at a different level in terms of his or her capabilities, and Krishnamacharya respected this and taught his students to do the same. Just as we teach a child first to crawl, then to walk, and only after these steps have been mastered, to run, we need to lead the student one step at a time towards his or her goal. Sometimes the steps are larger, sometimes they are smaller. Again, it depends on the student.

For the adults, including members of the Royal Family, who came to him for *cikitsa krama*, or healing, he carefully utilized all of the many tools of yoga to help alleviate their specific problems. He also used certain aids or supports for people who were limited physically. Many have since built on Krishnamacharya's method of utilizing special supports, which in today's yoga parlance are called "props."

People would approach Krishnamacharya, not just for physical or psychological healing, but also for spiritual healing. In such cases, he always took care to learn about the student's spiritual and religious beliefs before attempting to work with them. He believed strongly that we must not impose our beliefs on others, particularly in the areas of religion or spirituality, which are very personal. Also, each tradition's distinctive images and teachings may be precious to one, but not to another. When working with a Muslim student, for example, he would teach him to meditate on *Allah*. If the student were a Christian, he would ask her to meditate on *Christ* or *Mary*. He would never have given a devotee of Lord *Ganesha* the focus of *Mary* or *Allah*, because such images would probably have had no meaning for that person or may even have offended them.

In the case of a student who was a nontheist, he would never talk about God in their practice. Instead, he would ask them to meditate on things in nature like the sun, or the moon, or a mountain. One of his students, a Western Christian, asked Krishnamacharya to teach him the *mantra* on *Narayana*, one of the supreme Gods in India.

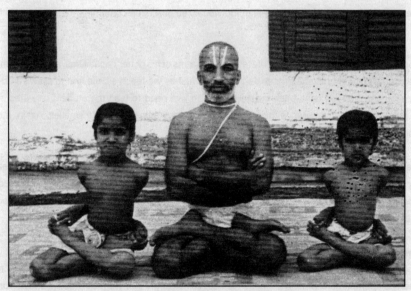

Krishnamacharya with his first two daughters doing *asanas* in the 1940s.

"*Narayana* is from my culture and tradition," Krishnamacharya told him. "You must find your own *Narayana* from yours. Only then will it work."

The student was extremely touched by this answer.

"Religion or spirituality is a personal practice. One must never impose it on another, unless the other seeks and is eligible for the same," was Krishnamacharya's strong opinion on this issue. Because of his respect for each student's personal spiritual practice, he gained the trust of people from many different backgrounds. He understood that the role of the teacher was to guide the student to discovery of his own spiritual path. The teacher must not impose that path on the student, because then the teacher would be asking the student to commit to something in which she did not believe. This not only renders the healing process less effective, it could have a negative impact on the student and would likely destroy the bond of trust between the student and the healer.

At this point in his career, with a successful, respected yoga school and a family of his own, Krishnamacharya could have settled in and enjoyed his life. But that would not have fulfilled his teacher's instruction to spread the message of yoga. So, Krishnamacharya continued traveling with his students to cities and towns all over India giving lectures on yoga and its benefits.

The depth of Krishnamacharya's wisdom and the amazing skill of his students captivated audiences, and also left them feeling a need to look more closely into their own cultural heritage. BKS Iyengar shared this impression of his teacher in a 1991 interview in the magazine, *Darsanam*. "T Krishnamacharya was endowed with a fine and strong body. There was a luster in his eyes and body. He had a strong mind. I was too young and immature to study [with] him and [understand] his capabilities. The ethos around my guru, his learning, deep insight, and experience made him stand apart from other masters."

At the end of these lectures, people often rushed up to Krishnamacharya and asked to become his students. He asked two things in return for instruction: that they spend a reasonable amount of time to undergo the training, and that they commit to their practice. He would remind them that knowledge was not obtained by studying the teachings, but by practicing the teachings.

Even in the midst of his ongoing work at the *Yoga Shala* and his busy lecture schedule around the country, Krishnamacharya always found time to garden. He would prepare the manure himself and take expert care in growing the trees and herbs. Most of the medicines that he prescribed to his students, he prepared at home using plants he had grown himself. This has always been the practice of the ancient teachers and the *Ayurvedic* doctors. Sadly, today the herbs and other ingredients used in *Ayurveda* are typically mass-manufactured, a manner of preparation which is contrary to the very foundations of *Ayurveda*.

Krishnamacharya's life, despite his growing renown and the respect and support of the King, remained simple, humble, and independent. Many times, the King would try and offer him more payment by sending a basket full of fruits in which he would have hidden some precious jewels. My grandmother told me how Krishnamacharya always had an uncanny sense about these things, and he would send the untouched basket back with the Royal Guard, along with a message to the King: "Sire. Thank you for these fruits. But I am afraid I cannot accept them as they have come with a set of thorns."

It disappointed the King that Krishnamacharya would not accept these gifts, but his affection for and trust in the yoga master only grew with each passing day. He consulted Krishnamacharya on many occasions. Even when he had to select a horse for his personal use, he would ask Krishnamacharya's advice, wanting to be sure the horse he had chosen was the right one for him.

Many others also approached Krishnamacharya for advice. In 1930, a public dispute broke out in Mysore between two religious traditions. A priest from the *Maharaja's* Sanskrit college was planning a *vajapeya yajna*, a ritual performed for the welfare of society. This ritual included the sacrifice of an animal to appease the Gods and earn their protection. According to the scriptures, animal sacrifice was permissible when it was done for the greater good, but when the *Jains* and the *Lingayats* (two sects of people living in Mysore) heard about this ritual, they were furious. Both religious sects believe in absolute *ahimsa* (non-violence), and they quickly formed an opposition group.

The district police commissioner, caught in the middle of the conflict, sent an urgent message to Krishnamacharya through the *Maharaja's* private secretary, asking him to come and ease the tension. Krishnamacharya went to the place of the *yajna* and called for both sides to come together for discussion. After a long debate, Krishnamacharya prevailed in his argument that there had to be a minimum amount of violence in order to sustain normal life. The *yajna* was performed, and there was peace in the region.

Krishnamacharya wrote a book, *Sastriya Yajna*, about the issue of sacrifice hoping to provide people with guidance on the subject and make them aware of the textual and philosophical basis of his arguments. Various institutions around Mysore also invited him to speak about this subject. His lectures drove home the point that, although sacrifice is essential in some cases, it must not be performed blindly, but only when it is the right *dharma*.

Krishnamacharya's travels in Mysore and around India eventually brought him to the attention of Western doctors and scientists. People outside of India were beginning to hear stories of the extraordinary powers of the Indian *yogi* who could stop his own heartbeat.

Professor Wenger of California and Dr. Therosse Brosse of Paris contacted Krishnamacharya in 1935, hoping to test the validity of some of these stories they had heard about *yogis* performing miracles. Krishnamacharya agreed to work with them. In the presence of other scientists attending as witnesses, he demonstrated to Professors Wenger and Brosse that both the mechanical and electrical actions of the heart could be modified at will. He also proved that he could pause his heartbeat for over two minutes. This experiment was conducted on January 23, 1936. The testimonial from Dr. Brosse mentions that ". . . not only has he proved beyond possibility of doubt that both the mechanical and the electrical action

.... record here our indebtedness to Mr.
Krishnamacharya, for the very kind help he has ......
us in our research work. We came here to read
with delicate instruments of measure the action of the
will upon the respiratory & circulatory functions.
Mr Krishnamacharya submitted himself to the
conditions of the experiments, and more than satisfied
our expectations. In fact not only has he proved, beyond
possibility of doubt that both the mechanic, and the
electrical action of the heart could be modified ......
which the West does not consider possible, but he
has enabled us to lay the foundations for a deeper
analysis of the yogic states than we foresaw.

        Our heartfelt gratitude remains with him and
with his helpers.
        Mysore, Jan. 23t, 1936.

Emile Kareault.   Brosse
.... Professor of Psychology.
& Square Rapp   Docteur Thérèse Brosse
    Paris (7) France.   in summer = 29 Boulevard ....
                           (may - october)   Royat (Puy de Dôme)
                                                France
                           in winter = 55 faubourg S. Honoré
                           (october - may)   Paris   (8)

The testimonial from Dr. Therosse Brosse, June 23, 1936.

Dr. MEHERWAN JEHANGIR, I. M. & S., I.C.P.S.

Dr. RUSTOM JEHANGIR, I. M. & S

HYDERABAD-DECCAN.

16th August 19 38

No. Cf. 26/335./b

This is to certify that SRIMAN VIDVAN KRI-
SHNAMACHARAY during the YOGA performance held at t
the YOUNG MEN'S IMPROVEMENT SOCIETY HALL on Friday
the 5th August 1938, was very satisfactorily able
to stop the beating of the Heart for a period of
more than two minutes, as heard by auscultation.

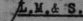

L, M, & S.

R/s.
erf.

Another testimonial from Dr. Jehangir, proving that Krishnamacharya stopped the heartbeat more than once.

of the heart could be modified at will, which the west does not consider possible, but he has enabled us to lay the foundations for a deeper analysis of the yogic states than we foresaw."

Krishnamacharya recollected that one man, a specialist from Germany, said after the demonstration, "I would have pronounced him dead."

Throughout India, thanks to Krishnamacharya's tireless efforts, people were beginning to pursue yoga more seriously, and not only because of these "miracles," but because the benefits were clearly real.

Krishnamacharya was also causing a stir in the country by teaching yoga to women. At the time, it was considered inappropriate for a woman to be taught yoga and other special teachings.

The reasons behind this are mentioned in the *Yoga Rahasya* of Nathamuni. Women, the text states, are more prone to gossip than spiritual practice. If we take this literally, there appears to be a contradiction in the text itself, because, in an earlier chapter, Nathamuni strongly advocates the practice of yoga by women. My feeling is that the reasons for not allowing women to learn yoga were actually far subtler. In those times, people lived very differently. India was under constant threat of invasion, the men often went into the forest during the day to pursue their practice or hunt for food, and women remained at home alone together, taking care of children, looking after the cattle, or working in the garden. So women were always in the company of other women, and this gave them an opportunity to talk about various things, including, the early masters concluded, their own practices, which were meant to be secret. This is probably why women were not taught many of these special practices, and why later masters enforced this custom and barred women from learning and practicing yoga.

But Krishnamacharya believed that women needed the peace of mind yoga offered just as much as men. He also recognized that women were going to play a leading role in modern society, and he believed that yoga would be of great benefit to them. The first women to whom he taught yoga included his wife, Namagiriamma, and his sister-in-law, Jayaammal. By 1936, Krishnamacharya already had three children: Pundarikavalli, his first daughter, born in 1931, Alamelu, his second daughter, born in 1933, and Srinivasan, his third child and first son, born in 1936. He taught all of them yoga, including his daughters.

Then, in 1937, a visitor arrived at the Palace of Mysore. The visitor was a foreign lady who had come to the palace with her husband, a close friend of the *Maharaja*, to attend a Royal wedding. When the lady heard about the yoga classes being taught at the palace, she asked the King if she could attend, and the *Maharaja* asked Krishnamacharya to teach her.

Krishnamacharya was skeptical of the lady's intentions and interest, and he replied that he would teach her, but only if she agreed to certain conditions. He instructed her to eat only certain foods and fruits and to finish her practice before sunrise, and then repeat the practice before him in the evening.

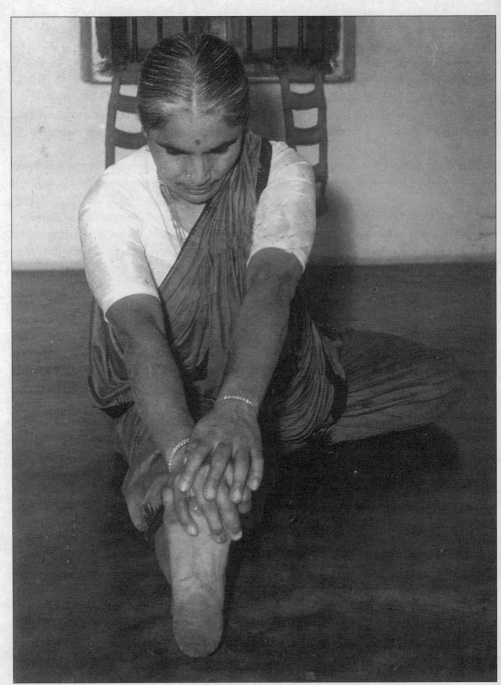

Krishnamacharya's first known female student, his wife, Namagiriamma, seen here practicing in the 1970s.

These were terrible conditions to ask the woman to meet, considering that she had come for a wedding, which would be accompanied by a lavish feast. Even before the wedding, there were many festive evenings filled with cocktails and dancing until the wee hours of the morning, but the lady had to retire early to finish her practice before sunrise, so she missed all of these pleasurable evenings. She faithfully followed Krishnamacharya's instructions and did not miss a single day of yoga practice. This pleased Krishnamacharya a great deal, and soon, he eased her conditions and she became a very special student of his.

The foreign lady's name was Indra Devi, and she became one of the most dynamic yoga masters of our time, taking yoga far out of India to countries such as China, the U.S., and Argentina, among many others. She kept in close contact with her teacher right up until his death.

I wanted to interview Indra Devi for this book, but, sadly, she passed away in 2002 before my letter reached her. I attempted to gather information about her relationship with Krishnamacharya from other sources, but I was unable to locate much in the manner of first-hand knowledge. Then, a dear friend of mine from Los Angeles, Larry Payne, came to my rescue. In the early '80s, he had organized a convention on yoga honoring Krishnamacharya's teachings. Both my father and Indra Devi participated in this convention, and Larry recorded everything on video. He generously offered to send me a copy of the video to use as a resource for this book.

I listened to Indra Devi speak passionately about yoga, her journey, and mostly, her teacher. One anecdote she related particularly impressed me. There is this idea in some yoga circles nowadays, that we have to force ourselves into a posture. But what Indra Devi relates about her practice and the teachings of Krishnamacharya defies this idea.

"I remember in one of the classes in the beginning, everybody was doing *Pascimatanasana*. Well, almost everybody. You know [the posture where your] feet stretched on the floor, and inhale—exhale you touch the toes. My hands were so far from the toes that I asked one of my co-students to push me from the back. *Sri* [Krishnamacharya] told me, 'No, no, no! You can injure muscle. You can do it by and by.' And I remember I'm on the floor, looking up at him and saying, '[maybe I can do it] in my next incarnation.'"

To me, this is a message at the heart of yoga's teachings demonstrated here so simply and powerfully by Krishnamacharya.

"Yoga," he always emphasized, "must be modified to fit you, not the other way around."

Krishnamacharya's reputation as a healer was spreading throughout India. Part of his extraordinary effectiveness as a healer came from his thoughtful combination of the teachings of yoga with those of *Ayurveda*, which he had learned from a great master called Krishnakumar, in Bengal. The traditions share similar teachings, and it is believed that Patanjali was the creator of both Yoga and *Ayurveda*.

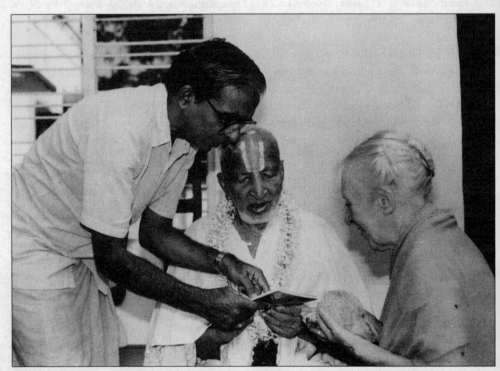

Krishnamacharya's first foreign female student, Indra Devi, seen here with her teacher and Desikachar.

Krishnamacharya's mastery of both disciplines allowed him to offer a more efficient and complete healing treatment to people with many different kinds of problems. If someone came to him with a liver problem, for example, Krishnamacharya would not only recommend yoga practices to address the sickness, but also suggest appropriate *Ayurvedic* preparations. Because he was a master of both schools, he could combine the traditions safely and offer a more effective treatment.

For Krishnamacharya, healing was always the most important aspect of his work. He believed that when people are not healthy, they cannot carry out their responsibilities in life. This is why he insisted that his students and patients practice every day. The power of yoga comes through only when there is daily practice. Krishnamacharya himself never failed to perform his own daily practice. His personal practice was precious to him, especially as a healer. If we as healers are not healthy, he contended, how can we heal other people?

On a recent trip to Sweden, I met with a friend of mine who is a psychoanalyst. We were talking about the most common problems experienced by people in Sweden. In the course of our discussion, my friend told me that the number one problem in the winter season in Sweden was depression. So, winter was also one of the busiest times of the year for psychoanalysts.

I asked her if I could test a hypothesis of mine.

"Sure," she replied without any hesitation.

"How often do you go for evaluation yourself?"

After thinking this over for a moment, she answered, "Once a year or once in two years, which is usual here."

"Is it at all possible," I said to her, "that you guys may get depressed because of the winter?"

"Surely," she said. "Sometimes even more than the patients, as we see one depressed patient after another all winter."

I pursued my hypothesis. "Do you think it's possible that when a patient comes to you, you offer treatment when you yourself are depressed?"

She had not anticipated this question, but being very honest, she answered candidly. "It definitely happens sometimes—not just with me, but with some of my other colleagues, as well. This is why I do yoga each day. It keeps me peaceful and calm and refreshes me each day so that I can be more attentive while at work. This is why yoga is so much better [than psychoanalysis], because you do your practice each day, and hence are evaluated each day. While in analysis, we are evaluated only once in a while."

It has been a particularly interesting hour I have had in discussing the subject of yoga & I am most favorably impressed with the rational explanations made by Prof Krishnamacharya. I believe him a thoroughly practical man.

G. A. Bernard
Los Angeles, California
24/10/36

An entry from the visitors' book of the *Yoga Shala* in Mysore. This entry shows that visitors included people from as far away as California.

Krishnamacharya knew this about yoga, that it replenishes us, refreshes and calms us, and gives us space to examine our lives. This is why he insisted on a daily discipline, not only to keep us healthy, but also to allow us the space to evaluate our overall health. And this is why his teaching becomes even more relevant in our hectic, harried modern times.

Day after day, the number of people visiting the *Yoga Shala* at Mysore increased. Many came for individual treatment, having heard about Krishnamacharya's healing powers. Others came to be students, and some came to learn to teach alongside him. The influence and reputation of the *Yoga Shala* grew, and soon, its numbers included foreigners, as well as Indians.

At the request of the King of Mysore, Krishnamacharya visited the neighboring state of Hyderabad to teach the family of the *Nizam* (Emperor) of Hyderabad. Krishnamacharya taught the Royal Family, incorporating elements of their own Sufi philosophy, which he had learned while traveling in the Himalayas. Their trust in him grew, and he became a good envoy for the *Maharaja* of Mysore.

Eager to spread the message of yoga, the *Maharaja* continued to send Krishnamacharya to cities in and outside Mysore State. He visited Madras, Bombay, Poona, and other well-known cities all over India. His fame spread, and in every city he visited, he gathered more students to yoga.

On one such tour in 1938 to Poona, the special interest of VB Gokhale of Deccan Gymkhana in yoga led Krishnamacharya to ask his student, BKS Iyengar, to stay in Poona to train and teach. Iyengar would make Poona his home for the rest of his life and establish the now world-renowned Ramamani Iyengar Memorial Yoga Institute there.

In that same year, 1938, on June 21, Krishnamacharya's wife gave birth to their fourth child, a second son, TKV Desikachar. They named him after the great *Sri Vaisnava* saint, Vedanta Desikacarya.

It is tradition in India that the eldest member of the family (usually, the eldest male member) picks the name of each child in the family. In the case of Krishnamacharya's family, he was the eldest, and so he named all of his children. Often, when his wife was pregnant, he would dream about a particular God or sage, and this would be the basis for his name choice. His first son, Srinivasan, for example, was born after Krishnamacharya dreamed about Lord *Srinivasa*, who is hosted in Tirpati, one of the most popular temples in India. And then, before his second son was born, he dreamed of Vedanta Desikacarya.

In the early 1940s, Krishnamacharya continued with his intense schedule of traveling and teaching. In July 1940, His Excellency Roger Lumley, the Governor of Bombay, invited Krishnamacharya to teach yoga to him. In March 1941, the *Maharaja* of Baroda invited Krishnamacharya to visit. He stayed there for three months, instructing the *Maharaja* in *asana* and *pranayama* at Laxmivilas Palace. He also gave lessons to the Divan, VT Krishnamachari, the private secretary to His Highness Pagar, and to *Sriman* Mansingraosubrao Ghorpade, father-in-law of the *Maharaja*.

Prof T. Krisnama charya, Professor of Yoga is bringing out publications on matters relating to yoga and particularly to yoga Exercises. I have just seen the "first Volume of his "..........". He is Keen on bringing out further Volumes. Needless to say he wants finance before he can do so. His venture deserves support and I hope sufficient encouragement will be forthcoming.

K.C. Lengakraya Reddy

7/6/50.

Chief Minister

Another entry from the visitors' book. This one is from the Chief Minister, who ordered the closing of the *Yoga Shala*. Here, he acknowledges the good work of the *Yoga Shala*, but is noncommittal of support.

Krishnamacharya's third son (his fifth child) was born in this same year. Krishnamacharya dreamt of the great Ramanujacarya, another *Sri Vaisnava* master. Ramanuja wrote a book called *Sri Bhasyam*, a commentary on the *Vedanta* teachings, and so Krishnamacharya named his last son, Sri Bhasyam.

By 1946, Krishnamacharya had received offers to teach from institutes all over India, including an invitation from the Ayurvedic Research Institutes hoping to enlist his guidance and support. He was also invited to Madras to help build yoga into the curriculum of the Ayurveda colleges. Meanwhile, the Medical college at Mysore sought his guidance in obtaining more information on the yogic system of physical education. Dr. Laksmipathy, Board of Studies in Indian Medicine, Madras, invited him to help them frame the syllabus dealing with *Ayurveda*.

By this point in his life, Krishnamacharya had achieved a great deal. He had managed to revive interest in the teachings of yoga, not only in Mysore, but in most parts of India. People from all over the country were reaping the benefits of yoga and its teachings, and they were eager to learn more. Through his travels, teachings, lectures, demonstrations, and healing practice, he had sparked a revival of the yoga tradition. Without the generous support of the *Maharaja* of Mysore, this would not have been possible.

However, this support was about to be taken away. The political landscape of the country was destined to change forever when India gained its independence from British rule in 1947. The powers of the local rulers were cut, and the *Maharaja* could no longer support the projects he wanted to support, projects like the *Yoga Shala*. The newly appointed Chief Minister of Mysore did not consider yoga important, and he immediately ordered the school closed within three months.

The students of the *Yoga Shala* organized a protest in front of the Chief Minister's house. Rushing out to meet them, the Chief Minister fell down the stairs and hurt himself. No one could cure him, and finally, Krishnamacharya was summoned. The Chief Minister was so amazed at the success of Krishnamacharya's healing treatment that he tried to reward the yoga master with money.

Krishnamacharya rejected the money, saying, "I don't want money. If you want to thank me, help the students of the *Yoga Shala*." But this was not a part of the Chief Minister's appointed agenda, and due to lack of funding, the *Yoga Shala* was shut down in 1950.

Krishnamacharya was nearly sixty-two years old with five children. He could have retired then and led a quiet life, like so many men of his age did. But that was not his intention or his goal. He had lost funding from Mysore Palace, but he had not lost the blessings from his teacher or his own zeal for his mission.

The golden days were far from over. They were just beginning.

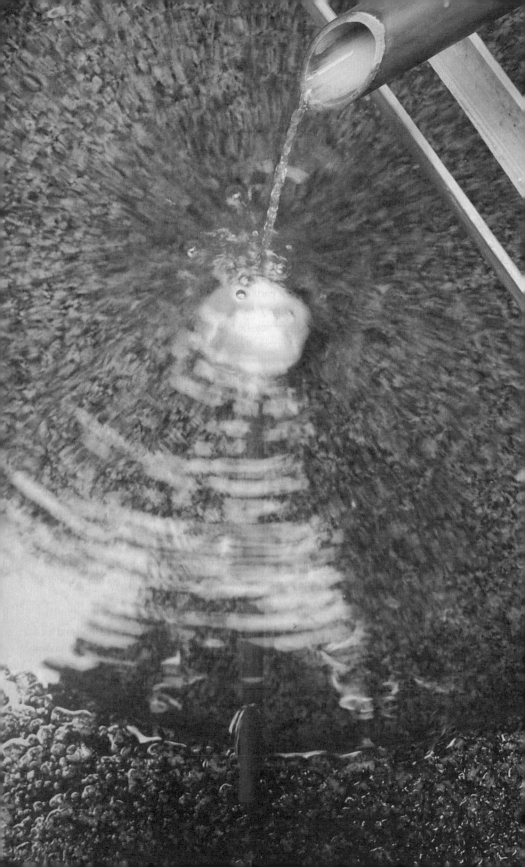

Chapter Six

Right Package, Right Delivery
the art of personalizing yoga

a fool thinks that there are two ways to do things:
his way or the wrong way.

"There is a problem," Jane* said quietly on the other end of the telephone. "I am having trouble with the practice you gave me."

Jane is a yoga teacher, and I have known her for many years. The last time she visited India, she came to see me about problems she was having getting a good night's sleep. After a thorough consultation, I drew up two practices for Jane to help her sleep better. One practice was to be performed just before sunrise, and the other, just after sunset. When she came to see me after her first day of practice, she was beaming, "Thank God. I slept like a baby last night. I am so happy."

I knew Jane to be a sincere and dedicated student, so I was concerned (and my pride was also a little wounded) when she called a few months later to say that she was having a problem with her practice.

"What is wrong Jane? Why is it not working?"

"I don't know. I am doing exactly what you told me to do. Exactly what I did in India."

I was perplexed. What could have gone wrong? I asked Jane if the temperature where she lived was very cool compared to the temperatures in India.

"It's summer here right now," she told me, "and it's quite warm."

"How long does it take to practice?" I asked her.

"Same time as in India. However, there is hardly any time between these two practices. I am not able to sleep enough, and I am not able to sleep during the day."

I was completely confused by now, but I persisted with my questions, and soon, the reason Jane's practice was no longer working for her became quite clear.

Jane lives in Sweden, and in the summer, the sun rises very early and sets extremely late. So when she performed her practice just after sunset, she was actually doing it very late, almost on the morning of the next day. Then just a few hours later, just before sunrise, she had to wake up to do her other practice. Jane was only getting a couple of hours of sleep each night. This was why her practice was not working for her anymore.

This incident is a perfect illustration of how the tools of yoga can work for us or against us. Every major yogic text talks about the importance of choosing the right yoga tools for any practice. In the *Yoga Sutra*, Patanjali discusses choosing the right tool and integrating that tool into the student's practice in an appropriate way, taking into account the student's needs, abilities, and situation.

---

* Not her real name.

tasya bhumisu viniyogah | Yoga Sutra III. 6

these appropriate [practices] must be applied considering the level where the student is

This is a classic *sutra*. Here, Patanjali introduces an amazing concept called **viniyoga**. The word *viniyoga* means "proper and continuous application." In the context of our yoga practice, this means the tool or set of tools used must be appropriate for the student, taking into account the student's situation, needs, and abilities, which may change over time.

For example, when an infant is born, the first food we introduce to the child is mother's milk. Later, we offer the baby food that is simple to digest, such as rice cereal or mashed bananas. Only later do we introduce solid, more complex foods. This is *viniyoga* in action. We choose the proper tool at each stage, and we refine that tool as the student progresses, just as in the case of the growing child. A teacher does not fixate on one tool and insist on applying it to the student when it is no longer beneficial, just as a mother would never insist that her child eat only mother's milk forever, nor would she feed a twelve-inch, deep-dish pizza to an infant.

Another example. When medication is given to infants, only a pediatric dosage is given. For an adult, the dosage would be different. Before prescribing medication to us, a doctor always takes into account any allergies or family history of disease. Also, we are asked to take medication only when we are sick, not when we are healthy. Western Medicine, then, also respects this concept of *viniyoga*—the proper and continuous application of the tools.

Again, just to clarify, the concept of *viniyoga* is not about the tool itself; it is about the appropriate utilization of the tool. And *viniyoga* is not just about choosing the right tool, it is about implementing it in the most appropriate way. *Viniyoga* is not a style or a type of yoga, it is the way yoga must be taught. Yoga will only work for us if we are given the right tools by a skilled teacher who knows how to utilize the tools in the most appropriate way for each individual student.

Jane's practice is a perfect example of the right tools utilized appropriately in one context, but when that context changed (context here referring to location), the tools were not only no longer useful, but they caused her distress. The tools I gave Jane were not appropriate for use during the summer season in Sweden. However, when she was doing the practice in India where the sun rises and sets at nearly the same time each day, it worked perfectly. In line with the principle of *viniyoga*, I refined her practice even more to make it an appropriate one for her, taking into consideration where she is living now.

Nathamuni's *Yoga Rahasya* also elaborates on personalizing each student's practice. In effect, this is the primary concern of the entire text. Nathamuni discusses how to teach yoga for people in different age groups, and why yoga should be taught differently to women, especially those who are pregnant.

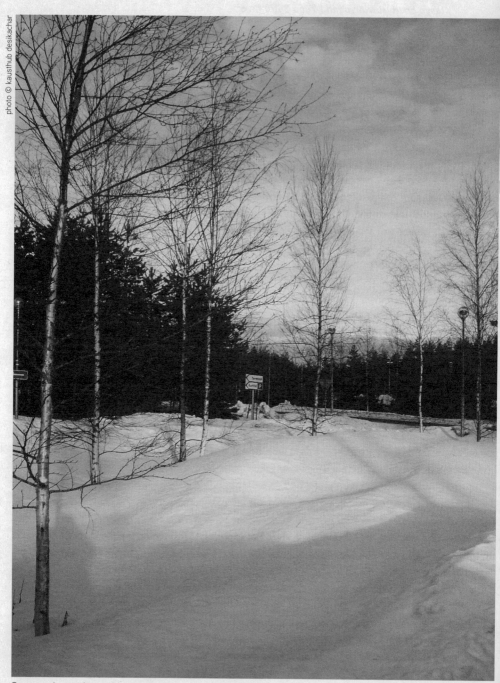

Seasons change the world around us. Also the world within us.

However, nothing is more useful than his discussion of the parameters a teacher must consider before she even decides what to teach to a student, which tool or set of tools to choose, or how to apply them.

kala: time

Time is the first parameter Nathamuni asks us to consider. This parameter has many dimensions, and each one is useful in determining the kind of practice to offer. For example, time could simply mean the time of the year. Consider the case of a country like Sweden, where the summer is so different from the winter that people even feel differently, depending on the season. Clearly, the time of year affects the human system, and so if I am going to choose a practice, I need to consider what time of the year my student will be practicing if I want it to be appropriate for him.

Kala could also mean how much time the student can devote to practice. If I am teaching yoga to a busy executive, and I insist that he practice two hours every day, he just won't do it, because he may not have the time. However, if I give him a fifteen-minute practice and ask him to practice twice a day or even three times a day, he may be able to manage it. And then, when he begins to feel better, he may decide this practice is good for him and precious enough and make more time for it.

Kala may also encompass time of day. Our body functions differently in the morning than it does in the evening. After a good night's sleep, we typically feel refreshed and full of energy, but the body may be stiff. In the evening after a long day's work, our muscles may feel more agile and flexible, but we are also tired. Hence, what we need in the morning may be different from what we need in the evening. This is why we need to respect the time of the day when deciding on the right practice.

desa: place

Desa refers to place and its influence on us. For example, some of us live in the mountains, others on the coast. In the mountains, especially if they are tall mountains, there is less oxygen, and often the humidity is much lower compared to coastal regions. This influences our system significantly, and we need to respect these geographic factors.

I remember once teaching yoga in Colorado to a group of people I have known for many years. I knew this group could easily do *pranayama* with long durations of inhale and exhale, so I introduced longer durations in their practice. Many of them told me they were finding this very uncomfortable. Their discomfort, I quickly realized, was due to the high altitude. We were nearly 6000 feet above sea level.

Desa also means respect for what the land offers to us. If I want someone to eat a particular kind of fruit as a dietary regulation, I must first make sure that this fruit is available in their area. If it is not, it would be impossible to ask them to follow this diet, even if I believed it would be the best thing for them. For example, if I recommend a totally vegetarian diet to someone who lives in Tibet, it will be difficult for them to follow it the entire year. At their altitudes, vegetables grow only three months out of the year, and Tibetans do not have access to grocery stores, so it would not be feasible to sustain oneself on that kind of diet.

vayah: age

Age is a very sensitive topic these days, but like it or not, from the day of our birth, we begin to age. There is no denying this fact. And during each stage of life we go through, whether we are children, adults, middle-aged, or senior citizens, our focus is different. Our resources at each stage—physical resources, psychological resources, emotional resources, etc.—are different as well.

When we are very young, our focus is on education, growth, and expansion of our mind's horizon. As adults, we are preoccupied with family and with social and professional obligations. As a middle-aged person, we begin to prepare for our retirement from professional life, while looking forward to spending time with our grandchildren. Our time as senior citizens is full of contemplation, introspection, and graceful preparation for the last stages of life.

The resources available to us at each of these stages are different, too. As youngsters and adults we have a lot of strength and energy, while, as we grow older, we have less energy and physical agility, but we have more time at our disposal. What we can do when we are younger, then, is very different from what we can do as we grow older. This fact needs to be respected, and this is why Nathamuni suggests that we take "age" very seriously.

vrtti: occupation/activity

Vrtti refers to the activity or job that we are pursuing at the moment. Vrtti is an important parameter, because it tells a lot about our state of mind and health. Many jobs these days are often a source of sickness, whether we realize it or not. For example, computer programmers who spend long hours staring at a computer are more likely to have eye problems than people who do not work under these conditions.

Also, asking a student about her job helps us determine the resources available to her. It can also tell us a lot about her lifestyle. For example, if we find out that a student works on a farm all day, it is reasonable to assume that he would be physically very tired by the end of the day, and so would need a rejuvenating practice, but not necessarily a physically draining one. On the other hand, if a student has been working behind a desk for years, then it may be okay to assume that she needs a dynamic practice that would improve the body's circulation.

These are just some of the ways in which inquiring into a student's occupation can help us personalize the practice we are going to offer the student. Today, in the era of specialization, this factor has become even more important.

sakti: strength/capacity

The next parameter that Nathamuni recommends we consider is the strength or capacity of the student. This includes not only physical strength, but also mental, emotional, and spiritual strength, and breathing capacity. Just as it would be unwise to ask a little baby to carry a heavy object, it would be inappropriate to perform any practice beyond our capacity. An inappropriate practice can lead to numerous kinds of problems. We must recognize our limitations and accept them with grace, instead of judging ourselves harshly and translating a limitation into a blow to the ego.

A student of my grandfather once read a book which claimed that if you hold after exhale for a long time, you will become slim. This man was quite bulky and desperately needed to lose weight, so he had been following the advice in this book, holding his breath after exhale for a long time. Very soon, he began sweating, and he could not control his urinary or bowel movements. It was a very embarrassing situation for him, and he rushed to my grandfather for advice.

When the man explained what he had been doing, Krishnamacharya said to him, "You nearly killed yourself by doing this. Your ability to hold your breath is very limited at this moment. You have pushed yourself beyond your ability, and this is why you are suffering. Don't ever do this again if you want to live healthy."

It took this gentleman nearly three months to recover from his problems.

It is clear that honestly evaluating strengths and weaknesses is crucial if we want to create an appropriate, safe, and beneficial yoga practice. This does not mean we must accept a situation that could be improved. The goal is to enhance strength step-by-step over a period of time.

Consider this example. When we were teaching a group of children with special needs at the KYM, we introduced them to some *asanas*. When we taught them *Trikonasana*, a twist posture, the kids could not get the movement right. They were unable to get the right hand towards the left foot, or vice versa. It would have been easy for us to give up and say, "Well these kids just can't do it." However, that would not have been the right approach. We have to respect that each child has mental strength.

One of our teachers came up with a brilliant idea to help the children find the pose. She tied blue and red bands on either arm of each child and tied a red and a blue band on the corresponding feet. She asked the children to bring the blue bands together, and then she asked them to bring the red bands together.

Bingo! It worked. Very soon each child's mental capacity improved, and they could all follow this movement without the help of the colored bands.

marga: direction

Marga represents our path, the direction we want to follow in life. Some of us want to become sportsmen, while others want to be philosophers. Some want to be healers, others want to work in public relations. Each of these paths requires a different set of skills and tools. Yoga can help us achieve our goals, and we can use it as a process of preparation. This is why we need to consider *marga* when devising a practice for a student. If the student has more than one goal, the focus of the practice must be on the most immediate goal.

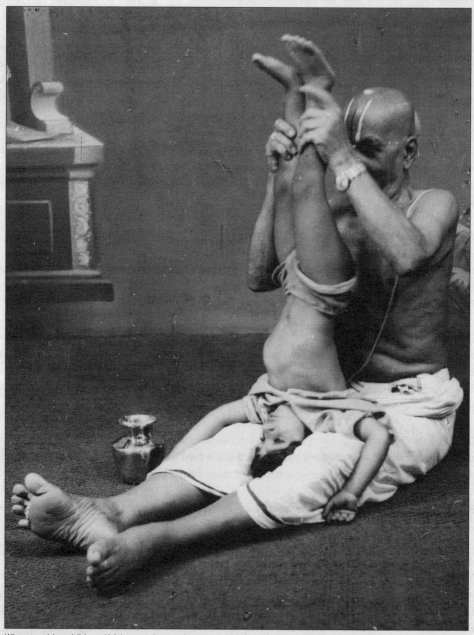

When teaching children, Krishnamacharya always made it fun. Here, he teaches his grandson Bhusan Desikachar.

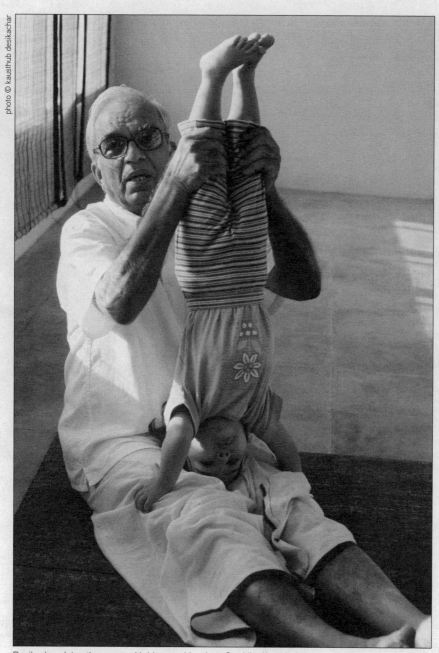

Desikachar doing the same with his granddaughter Sraddha Kausthub.

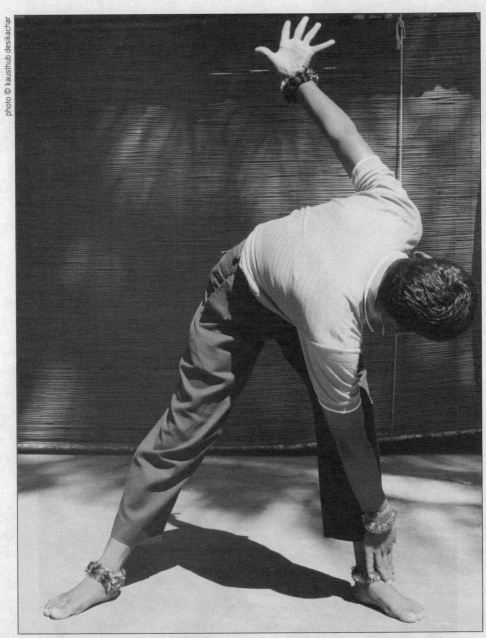

A special child being taught to do *Trikonasana* by bringing similar colored bands together.

A young boy named Ram was brought to my father because he reacted negatively to certain types of food and was in need of healing treatment. When my father met with Ram, one of the things he learned from him was that he was interested in rowing and wanted to take it up seriously. Even though my father was preparing a practice for healing the boy of his illness, he also introduced some physical movements that would enhance Ram's arm and abdominal strength and help him with his rowing.

It turned out that Ram's negative reaction to certain foods was due to a weak liver. To address this issue, my father drew up a practice for Ram that included certain postures like *Jathara Parivrtti* (Lying Twist). Gradually, he added sequences like *Surya Namaskara* (Sun Salutation) to strengthen the boy's body.

These sequences were introduced into Ram's practice in stages. In the beginning, the focus of the practice was improving the health of the liver, but as Ram's condition improved, aspects of strengthening the arms, shoulders, and abdomen were gradually introduced. Later, when his liver problem had improved significantly, the focus shifted to making him an expert rower. It's now a few years since we first met Ram, and not only has his liver problem been healed, but his rowing skills have improved thanks to the additional ingredients my father added to the practice.

When combining *marga* into the practice, we need to make sure that in introducing the secondary focuses, we are not taking away from the main focus of the practice. This is why my father addressed Ram's needs in stages, addressing his main problem first (sickness), and then he added postures to address the secondary issues.

The kind of intense, highly focused personalization of each yoga practice recommended by Nathamuni and Patanjali is quite different from the style of yoga being practiced in many studios and schools today. Yoga is being dished out in prepackaged, one-size-fits-all doses. Its rich tradition is being diluted, trivialized into various 'styles' based on how a posture appears or how it is done. All of this takes away from yoga's spirit and its power to truly heal and help us. How you perform a practice is not the main issue in yoga. It is what the practice does to us that is the most important thing. And the same practice won't have the same effect on every person, because every person is unique.

Imagine if everyone went to the hospital complaining of illness, and the doctor gave each person the same pill irrespective of individual problems, the ages represented, etc. That pill would not work for everyone, because not all of us suffer from the same problems, and we are all different in terms of age, physical condition, emotional state, lifestyle, personal history, etc. So each of us would require a different dosage, maybe even a different medication.

We are also different in terms of allergies and reactions. For example, some of us are allergic to certain chemical drugs. Hence, the doctor cannot blindly prescribe a drug, which may aggravate these allergies. Similarly, our medical history needs to be checked before treatment is offered. For example, a doctor will treat a patient with high blood pressure and a family history of the same very differently from a patient who has no such history.

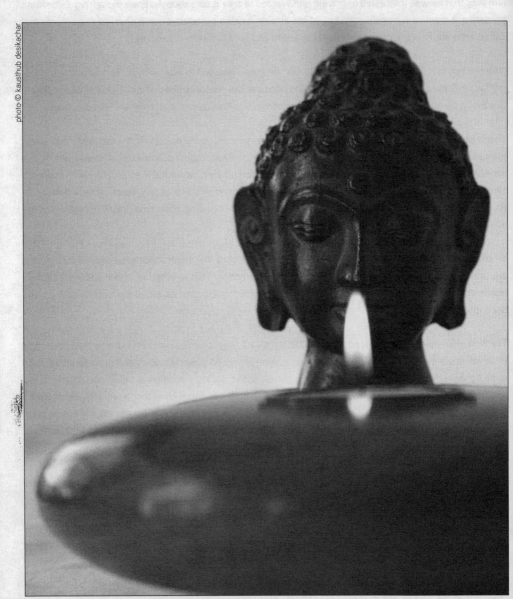

Respecting the uniqueness of every individual, even masters like the Buddha taught differently to each person.

It is the same when offering your students a "dose" of yoga. No one tool or set of tools will work for everyone. Nor will the same tool work the same way for every person. This is why the ancient yoga masters like Nathamuni and more recently, Krishnamacharya, personalized practices for their students that respected each student's strengths, honored their abilities, and addressed their needs directly.

Thanks to the wisdom of these masters and their teachings, I was able to get back to Jane with a more appropriate practice, one that would find acceptance even in the long days of the Swedish summer.

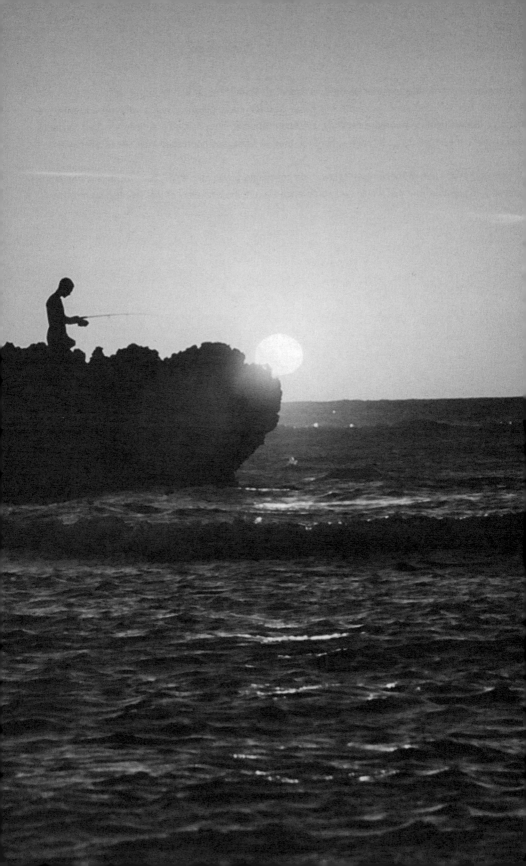

Chapter Seven

Destination Madras
the dawn of a new era

failing isn't as bad as not trying at all.
hope is the last thing we can lose.

By the time the *Yoga Shala* had closed forever, Krishnamacharya had five young children to provide for and no steady income. How would they eat? How would they continue going to school? The *gurukula* system had died out, schooling was not free, and Krishnamacharya had to pay rent on a home for his family. All of these expenses would have to be taken care of in some other way now that the income from the *Yoga Shala* was gone. I remember my grandmother saying that there were many days when Krishnamacharya ate very little or even nothing at all, so that his children would not go without.

Life was becoming more of a struggle for the family with each passing day. But Krishnamacharya still had his devoted wife, Namagiriamma, and his teacher's blessings, and neither had ever let him down. He was not discouraged by the thought of the challenges that lay ahead.

As it turned out, Namagiriamma had been very prudent, and during Krishnamacharya's tenure at the *Yoga Shala*, she had been setting aside money. The family was able to live off of these savings for some time, while Krishnamacharya traveled the country teaching. Namagiriamma ran the household so well while he was away that he did not need to worry about the welfare of his children, and he could focus all of his energy on teaching and earning money to support them. Krishnamacharya could always count on Namagiriamma to be a pillar of strength for him and for the children, especially during difficult times.

In 1950, Krishnamacharya received an invitation to teach yoga from Nageswara Rao, the owner of a large company called Amrutajan, which is still in operation today. The visit was meant to be a brief one, and he traveled alone to Madras while the family remained in Mysore, so that the children could continue their schooling. Rao kindly offered Krishnamacharya temporary lodging at his house.

Very quickly after he began working with Rao, word of Krishnamacharya's healing skills began to spread. Friends and associates of Rao asked Krishnamacharya to work with them, and he ended up prolonging his stay. He even rented his own single-room apartment in Royapettah High Road, opposite Madras Sanskrit college.

In this tiny, one-room lodging, Krishnamacharya practiced his daily rituals, did his yoga practice, treated patients, cooked, ate, and slept. When it was not possible to see a student in his apartment, Krishnamacharya would walk to the student's home. People in the neighborhood were amazed to see a man in his late 60s walk so fast and cover such long distances nearly every day.

Two of his sons, Srinivasan and Sri Bhasyam, joined him soon after he moved into the new apartment. Srinivasan, who had already learned some yoga, began assisting his father, and Sri Bhasyam, who was still very young, began his yoga training.

Krishnamacharya began teaching at the Vivekananda College at the request of the college's principal, Sundaram Iyer. The college was funded by the Ramakrishna Mission, which valued traditional Indian teaching. Krishnamacharya's class attracted many students, and in 1952, he was appointed Yoga Lecturer. He trained the students in *asana* and *pranayama*, and at the end of the term, they received a certificate.

It was in this same year that his last child and third daughter, Sri Shubha, was born in Chennai. By this time, Krishnamacharya's older children were beginning to move on with their own lives. His first two children, Pundarikavalli and Alamelu, were already married and living with their husbands.

It was around this time, as well, that a prominent Madras dignitary, TR Venkatrama Shastri, suffered an attack of paralysis. Shastri was a Senior Advocate and one of the top members of the legal council for the Tamilnadu State. Shastri's family had heard of Krishnamacharya's skills and asked him to help. Shastri's recovery over the course of therapy with Krishnamacharya was a revelation to many about the potential of yoga. His success in this case led directly to another important encounter.

The noted Jurist, Alladi Krishnaswamy Iyer, who had taken part in drafting the Indian Constitution, suffered a severe stroke that left him bedridden and unable to eat or speak. Krishnamacharya combined the best of yogic and *Ayurvedic* tools in a personalized treatment to help him. He prepared special *Ayurvedic* oil, which he would apply to his patient, and then, he would ask Iyer to do some simple *pranayama* practices. As Iyer's health improved, Krishnamacharya introduced simple movements to enhance mobility. After six months of careful treatment, Iyer could walk a few steps, communicate with people, eat on his own, and even hold a pen and write. Many people had believed it would be impossible for him to do any of these things again.

With so much work available to him, and with the encouragement of the community in Madras, Krishnamacharya decided to settle there permanently. He moved into a slightly bigger apartment, and in 1956, the rest of his family joined him (except Desikachar, who stayed on in Mysore to complete his university degree). A small screen separated the apartment into two rooms. One room was Krishnamacharya's teaching space, and the other room was the family space. It may not have been the most ideal living situation, but above all, the family was happy to be back together and move on with life.

This small apartment became the new headquarters for Krishnamacharya's mission. Here, he taught his students, wrote articles about yoga, and prepared medicines all from a tiny, makeshift room on Royapettah High Road. He also wrote a book here, **Yogasanagalu**. He wrote this book in Kannada, the language spoken in Mysore (today Karnataka State).

Literally translated, *yogasanagalu* means "yoga *asanas*." The book was an extension of his earlier book, *Yoga Makaranda*. In *Yogasanagalu*, Krishnamacharya classifies the postures into three categories: beginner, intermediate, and advanced. He also discusses how to determine which category is most appropriate for each student. There is a lovely introduction to yoga that explains the importance of *yama* and *niyama* in yoga practice, and Krishnamacharya also elaborates in this section on the concept of the *Astanga Yoga* of Patanjali. In the 1970s, Krishnamacharya would revise *Yogasanagalu*, adding a section on posture

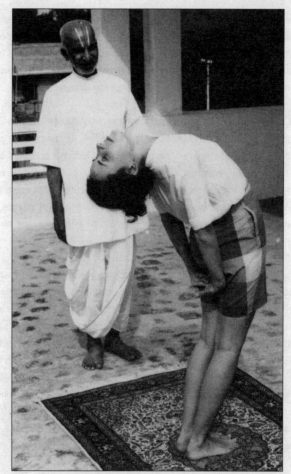

Krishnamacharya teaching *asana* modifications to a female student.

modifications. He had observed that the modern lifestyle was creating a less fit population, and it was necessary to offer more modifications in yoga classes because of this.

Long before Krishnamacharya set to work on the revised *Yogasanagalu*, however, the family moved into a larger apartment in Gopalapuram. This house had more rooms, including a nice verandah at the entrance. Now, Krishnamacharya could teach in a separate room, while the family shared the others. It was a much more comfortable arrangement for everyone.

The year was probably 1961, and Desikachar was home visiting his family. It was early in the morning, and he was reading the newspaper out on the verandah. Desikachar was an engineer by education and had just been offered a job in North India. He was transiting through Chennai on his way to his new job.

Suddenly, a huge car pulled up in front of their humble home. In those days, it was rare to see a car in Chennai, so when a very large one pulls up in front of your house, it's a shock.

Even more of a shock was the Western-looking woman in her fifties who jumped out of the car and ran towards the house shouting, "Professor! Professor!"

Desikachar wanted to get up and ask the lady who she was and explain to her that she was at the wrong house. Before he could act, however, Krishnamacharya walked out to receive the dignified-looking lady. The lady hugged Krishnamacharya and exclaimed, "Thank you! Thank you very much!"

Krishnamacharya led her into the house, welcoming her warmly. A perplexed and shocked Desikachar was left standing alone on the verandah.

It is still uncommon in India to see men and women touch each other affectionately in public. This is true even for couples. Of course, the younger generation is changing this, but in the 1960s, it was unheard of to see a man and a woman embrace in public. That is why Desikachar was so shocked; he had just seen a Western woman hug his very conservative father.

After Krishnamacharya bid farewell to the woman at the gate of their house, Desikachar asked him with a puzzled look on his face, "Who was that, and why was she hugging you?"

Krishnamacharya told him that the woman was a New Zealander. "She is Mrs. Malvenan," he said. "She has been suffering from insomnia. Last night was the first night in many years that she was able to go to sleep without taking a pill. Overcome with great joy, she came to thank me. I have been treating her for the past few months."

At that moment, something changed in Desikachar. He had heard about his father's healing abilities from other sources, but this was the first time he had seen the power of his father's work in action. He later recalls about the incident:

"I was amazed that this wealthy woman, who could afford the best Western medical treatments, was finding a cure with my father who was such a simple man, who knew no English or modern medicine. This is when I realized how great he was, and how great a teaching he had to share with people. It was at this moment that I decided to completely give up my career and become a yoga student."

Initially, Krishnamacharya was reluctant to accept his son's decision, but Desikachar's dedication to his studies soon convinced him.

In 1964, the family moved into a larger apartment in Mandavelipakkam. Now, there was enough space for all of them to teach. Many a student would benefit from the family of healers. With plenty of space available to him and his reputation firmly established in the area, Krishnamacharya's daily schedule of classes soon filled up, and he insisted that each student come for practice at his home.

Krishnamacharya's method of diagnosis was very systematic and accurate. A student rarely had to explain his problem in detail. Krishnamacharya would make his own observations and identify exactly what the problem was, sometimes simply by observing the student's pulse.

One of Krishnamacharya's students told me that Krishnamacharya always kept his eyes closed in class, but when a student made even a small mistake, he knew. His eyes would open immediately, and he would say, "Repeat once again."

Another student told me that he went to meet Krishnamacharya, and he had not been doing the practice Krishnamacharya had asked him to do. The moment he entered the room, Krishnamacharya said to him in a kind but firm way, "So, how is your practice this week? Looks like you have not practiced. Go home and come next week after you have practiced."

The practice Krishnamacharya created for each student varied, because each student was a very different person. He drew on all of the tools yoga has to offer to create a practice, he never depended on one tool alone. And he always made it clear to each student that this practice was exclusively for them and would not necessarily work for someone else. In every way, he respected the principle of *viniyoga* as presented by Patanjali and Nathamuni. Taking careful consideration of the time, place, age, occupation, capacity, and goal of each student, he designed unique practices to bring out the best in that person. He not only chose the best tools, he implemented them in the most appropriate manner.

For example, when Krishnamacharya taught children *srsti krama*, he taught it as though he were a child himself. These classes were full of energy, joy, and laughter. To hold their attention, he told the children stories about every *asana* and asked them to chant special sounds. He taught different postures each day, so that the children would not become bored. Best of all, at the end of class, he gave each child a sweet treat. I remember waiting in anticipation with the other children for him to hand me the sweet made out of almond and sugar.

The children's *srsti krama*-focused classes were very different from the practices he offered pregnant women. With a pregnant woman, Krishnamacharya was very careful and attentive, and he would communicate in a manner that increased the woman's self-confidence. He often taught expectant mothers special chants considered helpful during pregnancy, and he always explained the meaning of these chants to them. He would ask them to be very careful with their diet and lifestyle choices in order to protect their baby.

These are the qualities that made him a true teacher, a true *yogi*. Not only was he able to teach the right thing in the right way, he was also able to tell, through a very disciplined, keen observation, whether or not a student had been practicing in the right way. Probably, it was his own experience with his teacher and his practice of yoga each day that helped him develop such a fine sense about his students and the practice.

Krishnamacharya's own practice was very dear to him. He woke up very early in the morning, around 3:00 a.m., and did *asana* and *pranayama*. By 5:00 a.m., he had started his *puja* (worship) to his personal God, which was followed by chanting of the *Vedas*. He was very precise in his daily practice of the rituals. He never performed his rituals out of order or made mistakes in the coordination of the gestures and chants.

Before ending his morning practice, Krishnamacharya always placed the wooden sandals of his yoga master on his head as a gesture of humility and surrender to his teacher. For him, this was the most important part of his daily practice.

Morning classes began after breakfast, at 7:00 a.m., and continued until noon. The afternoon sessions began at 3:00 p.m. and continued until 6:00 p.m. The content of the classes varied. Krishnamacharya taught on different aspects of yoga and the yoga texts to many students, including his sons. His ability to shift with complete ease between one topic and another and one class and another many times throughout the day amazed those around him.

One class might involve a Yoga Therapy session, then in the next class he would teach the *Vedanta*, which would be followed by a class on *Ayurveda*, and then a class on Sanskrit Grammar, etc. Then, at 6:00 p.m., after classes ended, he performed his evening rituals. After that, he might work with a few more students or spend time with his wife and grandchildren. It was an amazingly full and busy schedule for a seventy-year-old man.

Whenever people tried to tell him how great or inspiring he was, or when they praised him he would gently but firmly stop them. "It is not me," he told them. "It is my teacher who is doing this. Without him I am nothing." This was not false modesty on Krishnamacharya's part, it was heartfelt humility before his teacher and the teachings.

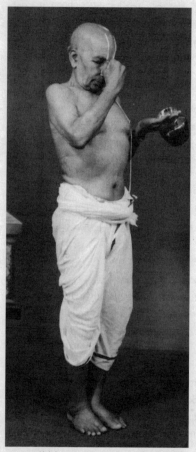 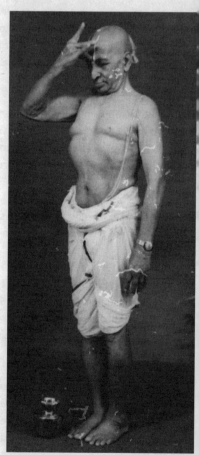

Krishnamacharya demonstrating two of the many steps in the daily ritual to honor and thank the sun.

n 1965, Jiddu Krishnamurti, the world-renowned philosopher and spiritual guide, requested an audience with Krishnamacharya after hearing of his skills from a student. Krishnamurti had been practicing yoga or many years, and he was looking for someone to help him with his personal practice. The men met at Vasant Vihar, the headquarters of the Krishnamurti Foundation in Madras.

Desikachar recalls this first meeting. "Krishnamurti had developed a lot of problems through his former yoga practice, which was inappropriate for his age and health status. This is why he sought a new teacher who could help him. One of his students recommended Krishnamacharya, who, he told Krishnamurti, was a great healer and yoga master. So Krishnamurti requested an audience with my father."

"My father took my brother Sri Bhasyam and me with him to meet Krishnamurti in Vasant Vihar. They had a pleasant interaction, and then Krishnamurti asked if he could see a demonstration of *asanas* and *pranayama*. My father guided me and my brother through some postures and breathing practices, which impressed Krishnamurti a lot. He knew he had found the right teacher, and he asked Krishnamacharya for help with his personal practice. My father offered to send me to teach him. He said would act as my guide, helping me to prepare and oversee Krishnamurti's practice."

Without hesitation, Krishnamurti accepted Krishnamacharya's offer, and Desikachar, guided by his father, began teaching him. Krishnamurti's condition and his practice improved with each passing day, and Desikachar and Krishnamurti became very close friends. On one occasion Krishnamurti told Desikachar, "I am going to offer you a scholarship. Even if it means I have to sell my shirt, I want to make sure you learn everything from your father. His great wisdom must not die with him." Desikachar and Krishnamacharya were touched, but they gracefully declined the offer. Krishnamacharya reassured Krishnamurti that everything would happen for the best, and that "what happens tomorrow is not always in our hands."

In May 1968, Desikachar was married to Menaka. He was thirty, and Menaka was a lovely girl of twenty-one. It was a traditional, arranged marriage. Krishnamacharya and Namagiriamma had chosen Menaka as a wife for their son. Desikachar was the first of the couple's sons to marry, and so it was also a special occasion; the first time a bride had entered the household.

My father recalled, "When I saw Menaka for the first time, she had come to our house with some of her relatives. My father and mother were talking to them, and soon they called me. When I came, this lovely woman was asked to prostrate to me. I assumed that my father was arranging for me to see a new student as he had done many times previously. However, after they left, he called me again and said 'you are going to marry this woman.' I was a bit taken aback that they were discussing my marriage, but I gracefully accepted. I am so glad now that I did."

The newlyweds shared the house with Krishnamacharya and the other members of the family still living at home. In the early 1970s, the entire family moved into a larger house in a neighborhood called Mandaveli. We still live in this house today. Desikachar bought the house with help from his father and some of his friends. He and Menaka lived on the upper level, and Krishnamacharya and Namagiriamma, along with Sri

Desikachar and Menaka during their wedding.

photo provided by menaka desikachar

Shubha, lived on the lower level. In 1970, the home welcomed Desikachar's first son, Bhusan. This was a very happy moment for Krishnamacharya, as Bhusan was the first child born to one of his sons.

Like the other houses, this house was a busy one. Krishnamacharya's mastery of so many different philosophical and practical topics drew scholars, politicians, artists, philosophers, and people of all professional and cultural backgrounds to him. They came for healing and also for advice and consultation on various teachings.

For example, Rukmani Devi, a renowned dancer and a scholar in the fields of art and culture, asked Krishnamacharya to clarify certain aspects of the *Ramayana* and *Mahabharata* for her, so that she could adapt them appropriately for her dance troupe. Soon, she also began taking yoga lessons from Desikachar. She was so pleased with the practice, that she asked Desikachar to teach yoga classes at Kalakshetra Academy, the famous dance school that she had founded. These classes stopped shortly after Rukmani Devi's death, but were revived recently through the Krishnamacharya Yoga Mandiram.

Krishnamacharya was also an authority in the field of astrology, and a particularly interesting case presented itself to him in the '70s. A young American friend of Desikachar asked Krishnamacharya to read his astrological chart. When the chart was brought to him, Krishnamacharya took one look at the man's face, then laughed and told the man that he was a born under the Pisces sign. This was not the sign indicated by the date of birth on his chart. Outraged at this remark, the man stormed out of Krishnamacharya's room. A few months later, however, he returned and said to Krishnamacharya, "Please forgive me, sir. You were right. I was born under the sign of Pisces. They made a mistake on my records when I was born."

It turned out that the nurse who filled out the records was a European immigrant who had fled to America during the war. The way Europeans (and even Asians) write the date is quite different from the format used by Americans. The mistake had escaped the notice of everyone, but it did not deceive Krishnamacharya.

Despite his fame and the praise and adulation offered by students and colleagues, Krishnamacharya never lost sight of his mission. He continued to teach and lecture and write poetry, essays, compositions, and texts on different topics in Yoga, *Ayurveda*, *Vedanta*, etc. By 1975, all of Krishnamacharya's children, except for Srinivasan (who remained a bachelor), were married. In 1970, Sri Bhasyam left the country and later married a French woman and settled in France where he and his family live to this day. Sri Shubha got married in 1974 and moved to Mysore, the home of her husband. This meant that only Krishnamacharya, his wife Namagiriamma, Desikachar, his wife Menaka and their two children, including myself (I was born in 1975), remained in the house in Chennai.

Desikachar was fast becoming a respected yoga teacher in his own right, and he was committed to bringing the message of his father's teachings to all of India and the world. In 1976, he founded the Krishnamacharya Yoga Mandiram (KYM) to honor his father and carry on his work.

125

This was indeed the golden era. Father and son worked together as a dedicated team, bringing the work of the ancient yoga masters to students around the world. Krishnamacharya regularly visited the KYM to supervise the healing work done by Desikachar and his team and to give lectures and provide moral support. Meanwhile, Desikachar poured his heart into the KYM and its work.

Krishnamacharya also composed numerous poems on yoga during this period. *Yoganjalisaram* is a collection of thirty-two verses, which capture the essence of yoga. *Dhyanamalika* is a poem with thirty-four verses that illuminates the deeper meaning of meditative practices.

In the late 1970s, MV Murugappan, whose family runs one of the largest companies in India today, began meeting with Krishnamacharya for health reasons, and the two became great friends. Krishnamacharya loved Murugappan's simplicity and humility.

Murugappan owned many cows and would often bring fresh milk to the house for Krishnamacharya and later, for Desikachar. He carried this milk to the house himself, and personally presented it to his teacher.

One day his grandson asked him, "Grandpa, we have so many servants and drivers, why don't you send the milk through them? Why are you taking it yourself?"

"I am taking this to my teacher, and it is my *dharma* that I do it myself," Murugappan told him.

Acts like this touched my grandfather deeply. He recognized his own values in Murugappan's actions.

I recently met with Murugappan, and he told me another interesting story. Having heard that his teacher had spent a long time at Mt. Kailash, he desired to visit this place himself. So taking the blessings of his teacher, Murugappan traveled to Mt. Kailash with a group friends. When he returned, he went to see Krishnamacharya to tell him about his trip. He told Krishnamacharya that he had taken a dip in the holy lake, Manasarovar, which is at the base of Mt. Kailash.

Krishnamacharya asked him, "How many dips did you have in the lake?"

"Only one sir. It was so cold," replied Murugappan.

Krishnamacharya started laughing so loudly that it worried Murugappan, who asked him, "Did I do anything wrong?"

"You went all the way to Mt. Kailash and Lake Manasarovar, and you only had one dip. How many chances will life give you to go there again?" Krishnamacharya said.

Recalling this, Murugappan told me, "I never thought about it this way. He was right. I could have had at least one more dip in the lake."

When I asked him what he had taken away from this incident, he immediately replied, "This taught me to reflect carefully on how I conduct my life. For life does not give second chances."

The two men continued to meet often, and very soon Murugappan was bringing along his brothers, cousins, and nephew to work with Krishnamacharya. Over time, the families of Murugappan, Krishnamacharya, and Desikachar became close friends, and this friendship between the families continues to the present day.

In 1984, Krishnamacharya, who was ninety-six years old, woke up one morning at his usual time well before sunrise. In the dark, he went to the bathroom, and when he came back to sit where he thought the bed was, he fell to the floor and broke his hip. It was his practice to rearrange the furniture in his room according to the changing seasons, and he had forgotten that he had moved his bed the day before.

The injury affected Krishnamacharya's daily life dramatically. He could no longer move around with the same agility as before, and he lost a significant amount of his cherished independence. The accident profoundly changed his life and the focus of his personal, spiritual work.

But Krishnamacharya was not discouraged. He had absolute faith in yoga. He devised a practice for himself, which he performed for the next few months. Much to the amazement of his family and doctors, he was soon able to move well and even walk a few steps.

After this incident, Krishnamacharya arrived at the decision to withdraw further into himself. He moved out of the main house into a structure on the same grounds. Following the instructions of his *guru*, he did not renounce his family and take *sannyasa*, but he did move into a different space, physically and spiritually.

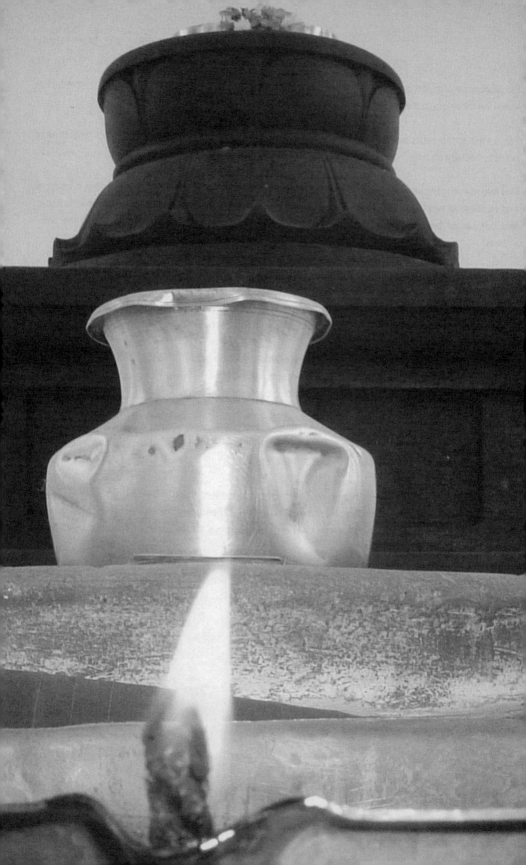

Chapter Eight

Why Yoga Works
the science behind the art

there are some questions that can be answered easily.
others, that can't, are the ones that are elevating.

"Help me, please!" cried the woman at the feet of the old man sitting on his couch.

The woman asking for help appeared to be in her late thirties, and she was clearly distressed. She was not one of Krishnamacharya's students, but she had visited him before as a companion to her sister, who was a student.

Krishnamacharya rose from his seat and said, "Please tell me what your problem is, and I will see what I can do."

Between heavy sobs, the woman, whose name was Shanti*, told Krishnamacharya that she was unable to conceive a child and this was destroying her marriage. Her in-laws wanted the family lineage to continue, and so her husband was threatening to marry another woman.

Even today in Asian countries, many families consider lineage vitally important. Continuity of lineage ensures the survival of family tradition, and if a problem arises that might endanger this survival, there are certain conventions in place to address this. In the case of a wife unable to conceive, the husband is allowed to remarry. If the husband were the source of the problem, the wife would also be allowed to remarry, although this is more rare.

In Shanti's case, after examining both her and her husband, the medical doctors found no reason why they should not be able to have a child. But in the eyes of Shanti's in-laws, none of this mattered. They pressured her husband to take action and protect the family's lineage. In desperation, Shanti had come to Krishnamacharya hoping for a miracle.

Reassuring her that he would try his best, Krishnamacharya asked Shanti to return in a week.

One week later, the woman returned. Krishnamacharya took her outside into the sunshine and recited a famous invocation of the sun. Afterwards, he presented her with a special powder wrapped in a clean leaf and said, "This medicine has been blessed by the sun, the giver of life. Each day you mix this with a bit of honey and consume it. Along with this, you must do the practice I give you. After thirty days, you must try to conceive the baby."

The woman gratefully accepted her magical medication and her practice and returned home.

In a few months time, Shanti returned to her teacher, joyful and excited. "Sir," she said, "it is now confirmed that I am pregnant. I want to thank you for getting rid of my illness. Without you, I would have suffered so much. I don't know how to express my gratitude for healing me."

---

* Not her real name.

130

Krishnamacharya smiled gently and replied, "It is not I who have healed you. It is your faith that has healed you. Had you not had faith in me or the practice, you would not have been healed at all."

Faith is one of two key factors that determine whether yoga will work for us or not. We may be offered the best techniques by our teacher, but if we have no faith in those techniques, in our teacher, and in the practice, then they will never work for us. Faith is the "magical" ingredient, intensifying and deepening the powerful work of yoga in our lives.

There is a word for faith in Sanskrit that Patanjali uses in the *Yoga Sutra*. That word is ***sraddha***. This word is a very beautiful word. Its root is *dha*—"to hold" or "to sustain." So the unfolding idea at the root of *sraddha* is that if we have faith, it will sustain us or hold us; faith will not allow us to fall or falter. According to the *Yoga Sutra*, when we have faith, we can achieve anything, even in times of great difficulty and suffering.

When Krishnamacharya tripped and broke his hip, my father immediately called for the family doctor. The doctor, realizing that Krishnamacharya had broken his hip, sent for a colleague, a specialist* in setting bones.

But Krishnamacharya was in no mood to entertain a host of doctors. The moment the specialist arrived, he demanded that all of the doctors leave. "I can handle myself and heal myself, and I will prove it to you within three months. I don't need your help," he told them with feeling.

Stung by Krishnamacharya's words, the specialist stormed out of our house. "Don't waste your time on a ninety-six-year-old insane man," he grumbled at my father. "He is not going to last long."

But Krishnamacharya had faith in his yoga, the yoga he had learned from his master. His theory was if he could heal at all, then yoga could help him heal even quicker.

Three months after the fall, Krishnamacharya called my father to his room and said, "Call that specialist." When my father telephoned the specialist and informed him that Krishnamacharya wanted to see him, the specialist responded with sarcasm, "So, now he wants me to come and help him."

When the specialist arrived, he was taken to Krishnamacharya, who greeted him and said, "That day [when I fell] you asked my son not to waste time on me. Look what I can do."

Krishnamacharya got up from his bed, walked a few steps, and then demonstrated for the amazed specialist a whole range of yoga postures that would have been challenging even to a younger, healthier person.

---

* At the request of the specialist, I have not used his name in this book.

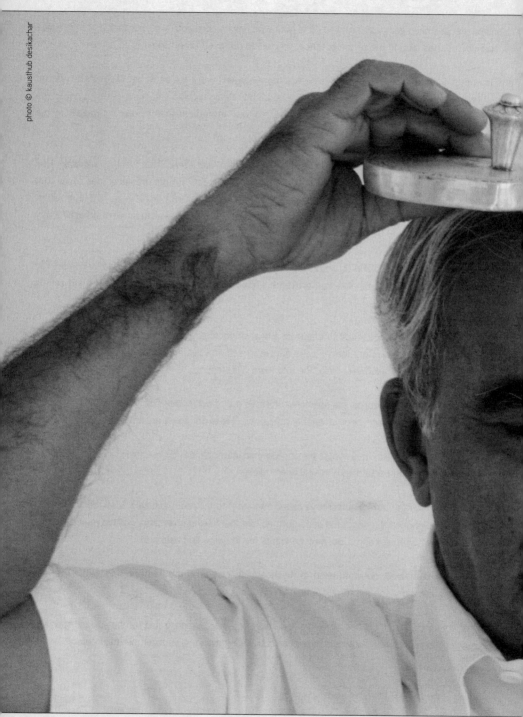

Desikachar demonstrating an expression of faith practiced since the time of the *Ramayana*. Here, the student places the sandals of the teacher on his head, reinforcing his faith in the teacher and the teaching.

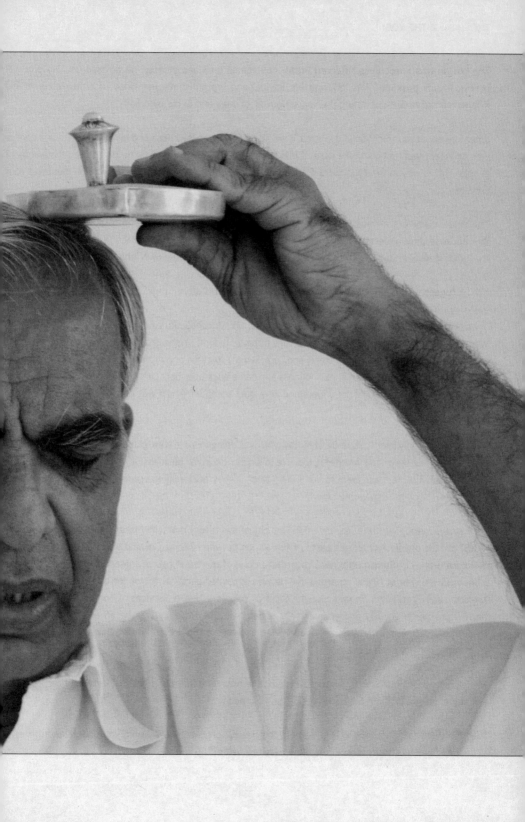

The doctor was speechless. "Record these movements on video please," he advised us. "No one will believe this is possible." We followed his advice, and we still have the video of nintey-six-year-old Krishnamacharya demonstrating the healing power of yoga and of his own faith.

When you are in your nineties and injured, it would be so easy to lose hope and faith. But Krishnamacharya was confident that he could take care of himself and heal himself. After all, he had healed thousands of people. This is why in the *Yoga Sutra*, Patanjali says that if you want to test your faith, you must test your confidence.

The ancient masters always tested the faith of each student before agreeing to teach them. They did this because they understood that if the student had no faith, then any practice they chose to teach that student would not work. The teachers did not want to waste their own time or the student's time.

MM Murugappan, the nephew of MV Murugappan, related this story to me.

"I was introduced to Krishnamacharya by my uncle, MV Murugappan, who was already a student of his. When I first met him and expressed my desire to be a student, Krishnamacharya asked me to come one week later. One week later, I was there, and he asked me to come one more week later. I thought that this was strange, but I accepted [his instructions] and came back one more week later. Again, I was asked to come a week later, [and] I did not understand why, but I accepted. And it was only this week that he began teaching me."

"I must say that only later [did I understand] why he was doing this. He was testing my faith and commitment before accepting me on this journey. I, too, use this ploy now in my business. If a person wants to seriously do business with me, I ask them to come back later. If they are really interested, they will come back. If not, I know I don't have to waste time."

I am always looking out for a way to test the validity of this theory that faith makes things work. In the mid-'90s, I had the opportunity to take part in a discussion between Desikachar and the late neurosurgeon Dr. B Ramamurthy. Dr. Ramamurthy was regarded as one of the finest neurosurgeons in the world, the first from India. He was so highly regarded that he was appointed personal doctor for almost all of our Prime Ministers and Presidents. He was also the Chief of Voluntary Health Services, an organization that offers health care to the socially and economically underprivileged. Not only was he an expert in the field of medicine, Dr. Ramamurthy was also well-versed in many of the ancient Indian philosophies and quoted from them with impressive ease.

My father and Dr. Ramamurthy were discussing the brain and its role in healing. I saw a chance here to ask some questions about faith and healing, so I jumped in.

"Sir, the *yogis* talk about the role of faith in the healing process. How would you understand this as a scientist? Does this really work? Does this have any value?"

Dr. Ramamurthy's reply solved the puzzle for me.

"Our body functions based on signals sent by the brain," he said. "If the brain sends a signal to the hand to move, it moves. If the brain sends a signal to the eye to open, it opens. Everything in our body happens based on the signals the brain sends. And these signals can be either positive or negative, and this makes a whole difference to how we are, and how we function. When we have fear, anxiety, etc., the brain sends negative signals, and this is why we feel the way we feel when [we are] overpowered by such feelings. However, when we have faith or confidence, the brain sends positive [signals] and this is what promotes healing. This is known in medicine as the placebo effect. Our ancient masters called it *sraddha*."

At that moment, I understood why the ancient masters placed such importance on the role of faith. Krishnamacharya healed people by igniting their faith. This is how he healed himself, and also how he healed Shanti. The magic medicine he offered to Shanti turned out to be nothing more than the ashes of a special kind of wood. But to Shanti, this offering was not "just" ash, it was something special from her *guru*, and she believed that it had the power to heal her.

Yet, as Krishnamacharya would tell his students again and again, in yoga even faith alone is not enough. **Self-empowerment**, the second ingredient in the healing process, is as important as faith.

The job of the patient in most systems of healing is to receive the treatment, and nothing more. Someone else performs the actual work of healing the patient. For example, we go to a surgeon, and he does the healing work while we are under anesthesia, unconscious and completely immobilized. While he is performing surgery, we don't even know what is happening or who is working on us.

Even when we take a pill our doctor has prescribed for us, the only effort we are expending to heal ourselves is remembering to take the pill and then performing the physical act of swallowing it. The pill does the rest of the job.

Similarly, when we go to a chiropractor, our role in the healing process is limited. The chiropractor works on healing the body for us. It is the same with massage therapy. When we get a massage, the therapist does the work, and we lie passively on the massage bed. Sometimes, we even fall asleep.

However, yoga is different. If yoga is going to heal us, we have to do the work. Yoga engages us directly in the healing process. We are active participants in our own healing treatment. As Krishnamacharya told one of his students, "It's no use to pray to God for help if you are not acting to help yourself."

Every major yogic text, including the *Yoga Sutra*, says the same thing. In yoga, in order to heal or to achieve any goal, the student needs to commit to the practice and have faith in the practice and the teachings. These requirements of discipline and faith are complimentary. If our faith is true, it will inspire us to do the things that are needed to move forward. Similarly, when we commit to our practice, approaching it with determination and eagerness, it will enhance our faith. Doing the work, having faith in the work, I am empowered, and I become my own healer.

Beyond commitment and faith, there is the practice itself, which, if it is to be appropriate, should possess certain qualities.

sa tu dirghakala nairantarya satkara adara asevito drdhabhumih | Yoga Sutra I. 14

the [appropriate] practice, pursued over a long time, without interruptions, with eagerness and positive attitude will indeed provide a strong foundation [to reach and sustain the goal]

Patanjali tells us about these qualities in the *Yoga Sutra*. Once we choose the appropriate practice, he wrote, we must be patient and practice it for a reasonably long period of time. Yoga does not provide "quick-fix" solutions. Healing, in any of the forms in which we may seek it, takes time. This is why we need faith and commitment in our practice.

If we are not consistent in our practice, if we practice for a few days and then skip a few days, we send the body mixed signals. For healing to happen, we must send a consistent message to our entire system. This means we must be disciplined, and in order to be disciplined, we may have to give up certain things that lead us away from the practice. Maybe, we need to watch less television or cut short our sleep, so that we can practice. There is an element of sacrifice involved in committing to our practice. In yoga, this is called *vairagyam*. *Vairagyam* is about detachment and letting go. If we have no *vairagyam*, it will be difficult to practice successfully. Distractions will always come up and try to draw us away from our goal, but if we cultivate the quality of *vairagyam*, we will be able to find our way back to the path and continue moving forward on our journey.

Eagerness and a positive attitude are also essential elements in a successful practice. As Dr. Ramamurthy said, when the brain sends positive signals to the body, this aids the healing process.

Yogis would present this idea in a slightly different way, although, in essence, they speak of the same phenomenon. Eagerness and a positive attitude, a *yogi* would say, are signs of faith in the teacher or the practice. Conversely, if these qualities are not present in the student, there is a deficiency of faith and the practice won't work. Whichever way you choose to look at it, it is important that these qualities are part of our practice.

When we are committed to the practice, when we practice with eagerness, a positive attitude, and faith, the healing happens from within us, not outside of us. There is a powerful healing force within us, which the *Yogis* call *prana* and the Chinese call *chi*. When we are disciplined in our practice, we connect with and nourish this powerful force or strength. This connection facilitates the healing process, even in situations where it appears that healing may be impossible, as in the case of Steve, the Qantas flight attendant, who was paralyzed by a stroke.

What the *yogis* call the *prana*, the Chinese call *chi*, which they nourish through *tai chi huan.*

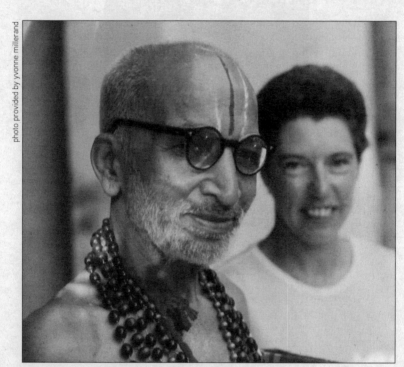

photo provided by yvonne millerand

Krishnamacharya always valued and nurtured good relationships, whether it was with students (above) or with others who walked through his life, as in the case of this photographer (facing page).

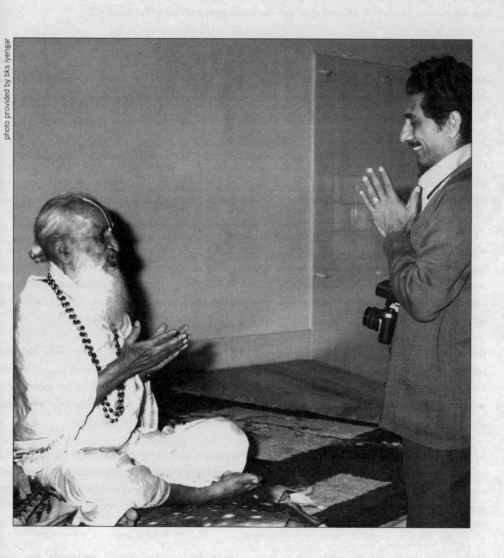

Only when he began to practice yoga, Steve told me, did he realize "that I had control over myself and what I do. And when this recognition came, I felt that I could take charge of my healing process."

A few years ago when I was just opening my eyes to the possibilities of yoga, I asked my father, "But how can we nurture this faith in people? How can we make them practice with discipline?"

My father did not give me an answer immediately. He only said, "You will find out yourself."

After many years of observing the way my father deals with his students, the way he communicates with them and inspires them, I finally came to the conclusion that the answer to this question is within each of us. If we do not have faith, how can we inspire faith in others? Would it be fair to expect another person to have faith, if we ourselves don't have it?

Only a person who has faith can ignite faith in others. Because Krishnamacharya had faith in yoga and demonstrated that faith many times by overcoming the obstacles and suffering in his own life, he inspired other people to have faith in yoga. If he had not been convinced of the power of yoga, it would have been difficult for him to convince others.

A good relationship between teacher and student also inspires faith. If I have a good relationship with my teacher, then I am more likely to have faith in her and listen to what she says. But if our relationship is problematic for any reason, then no matter how good the teacher is or how true the teachings, I will have trouble trusting that teacher. So as teachers, we must cultivate good and appropriate relationships with our students that inspire faith and trust.

One day, a family we are acquainted with brought their thirteen-year-old daughter to our center. The girl had cancer and had already gone through surgery and chemotherapy. These treatments caused her to lose all of her hair, including her eyebrows and eyelashes. She was very depressed about her appearance and worried that the other children at school would make fun of her. On top of this, the treatments had affected her hormones, causing excess bleeding during menstruation and enormous pain.

All of this was very traumatic for this young girl. The doctors gave her medications and recommended more treatments, but not one of them would take the time to sit and talk with her about her problems and concerns. They read the data in her file and offered prescriptions, and that was all. She hated going to the doctor now or to any healer, for that matter. Her parents were tense when they brought her to my father, worried about how she would react.

My father sat and talked to the girl for nearly an hour. He inquired about her school, her friends, what she liked to do, etc. He talked to her like a friend, played tick-tack-toe with her and told her riddles, but never once did he speak to her about sickness or illness. Before he left, he told her that he would see her the next day.

As my father was walking out, the father of the girl rushed up to him and asked him, "Sir, you have never asked her about her problem, nor have you seen her files. Why are you asking her to come tomorrow?"

My father smiled and reassured him, "Sir, I know your concern, but I assure you that it will be taken care of."

When the family arrived the next day, the mother told Desikachar, "Sir, for the last twenty-four hours [my daughter] has been talking only about you to everyone in the family. She has been counting the hours to get here and be with you."

When my father asked the girl the reason for this, she answered simply, "I like you. You are the only one who does not talk about my strange appearance, and the only one who has played so much with me."

Desikachar asked her if she wanted to play a little more, and she eagerly assented. He introduced some postures to her as a form of play and asked her to repeat them. She repeated them exactly as he had taught, and he offered her more. Then he told her that he would write down all of the postures on paper, and she should practice their game each day, so that she would become the best. The girl readily agreed to do as my father asked, and thus, began her yoga practice. She met with Desikachar every week and learned a new "game" which she would then practice at home.

A few weeks later, my father asked the girl if he could introduce some breathing into their game that would help her sickness. She agreed to his request without hesitation.

I met with the girl's father a few months later and asked him how his daughter was doing. He said to me, "I have never seen her happier. She loves her teacher. She practices her yoga every day without fail, even if she forgets to do her school homework. Her health is also much better. Her bleeding and cramps have reduced considerably. There is less trauma for her now."

This is an excellent example of the role the teacher-student relationship plays in yoga practice, and how it can inspire faith in the student. My father's first focus in working with this girl was to establish a good relationship with her, so that she would trust him and be guided by his words. Had he not built up this trust relationship with her first before offering treatment, she would never have come to like him or the practices he offered her.

But what if someone has no faith at all? Krishnamacharya believed that there is no one without faith. What each of us has faith in may be a different issue, but it is impossible to have no faith at all. Krishnamacharya, a cheeky smile lighting his face, would tell those who disagreed with him, "I have faith that everyone has faith. While you have **faith** that not everyone has faith."

Chapter Nine

Glorious Sunset
transitioning from one world to another

nothing is created nor destroyed,
it just changes from one medium to another.

The hip dislocation left Krishnamacharya with limited mobility. For a man who had been physically agile his whole life, this was a huge blow. But Krishnamacharya met this new challenge with grace and continued moving forward with life.

One of the messages of the *Yoga Sutra* is *Isvara Pranidhana*, or total acceptance of what is happening in our lives. Krishnamacharya practiced *Isvara Pranidhana*. He accepted his situation and went on with the business of living life. The fracture may have limited his mobility, but it did not affect him in any other way. After a brief rest, he began teaching again.

Krishnamacharya's recovery might not have been so quick or so successful without Namagiriamma's devotion and attentive care. During the time he was bedridden, she woke up before sunrise to prepare him for his day. Krishnamacharya had always been an early riser, but to help him maintain his schedule, Namagiriamma had to wake up even earlier to get herself ready, so that she could then focus her attention on him.

Krishnamacharya was very independent, but after he broke his hip, he had to depend on his wife's help with many simple tasks and activities. Sometimes, he became very frustrated over this.

I remember one such incident. It was during a particularly heavy monsoon season. A lot of water was accumulating in our streets, and the rain continued pouring down as if it might never stop. Water was rising and flowing into the compounds of every house on the street, including the children's school on the opposite side of our house.*

We have a two-storey house. My grandparent's bedroom was on the ground level, and my parents, myself, and the rest of the children were on the floor above. We knew that water was going to enter the ground level, and my father asked my grandparents to come upstairs, so they would not end up stranded in a room full of water.

But my grandfather refused to move from his room. My parents' and my grandmother's pleading could not convince him to come upstairs. My father and a student of his even tried to remove my grandfather from his room forcefully by carrying him out, but my grandfather was so strong even in his late nineties that they couldn't budge him. I remember my grandmother's tears when she realized that he was not going to leave.

"Go to sleep," my grandfather told her. "Everything will be fine in the morning."

That night the rain came down even harder, and I am sure that my grandmother and my parents did not sleep one wink.

---

* This was mainly due to the bad drainage system we had in those days. Things are much better now, thank God.

There was no sound from Krishnamacharya. At some point in the middle of the night, we all heard a loud thud, but nothing else.

When we woke up in the morning, the rain had stopped, and a surprise awaited us. There was no water in our house or anywhere on the street outside.

"See," my grandfather declared triumphantly, "I told you. Lord *Narayana* is on my side."

We went outside to find that the old compound wall of the school had collapsed, probably because of the extreme pressure exerted on it by the long, heavy downpour. Since the school was on a much lower level than our street, all of the water had drained into the playground instead of pooling in the streets and houses. I could see the relief on my grandmother's face.

My grandmother was committed to her role as nurturer and caretaker for my grandfather during this time, even though she was battling non-Hodgkin's lymphoma, a type of cancer that affects the lymphatic system. I remember accompanying her many times to the Chemotherapy Center, and even though she had very little energy on most days, she only let herself rest after attending to my grandfather's needs.

Yoga cannot possibly cure cancer, and Krishnamacharya knew this. He always emphasized that, "No one system has all the answers to all of our problems." He worked with my grandmother on a healing treatment, giving her *pranayama* and some meditation practices that would help heal her anxiety and distress and make her stronger. She would practice conscientiously, not only to take care of herself, but also to take care of him.

It is my strong feeling that her yoga practice is what allowed her to carry on with life during her last years. She was one of Krishnamacharya's oldest students (and most definitely the first female) and had been a sincere practitioner of yoga for a very long time.

Namagiriamma played a role in Krishnamacharya's recovery that went far beyond taking care of his mundane needs. He had always been a very independent man, but his injury forced him to depend on others for the first time in his life. There were moments when he would get very depressed, because he was not able to do things on his own, and he felt he was becoming a burden to his family, although we never felt this way. It was at these moments that Namagiriamma would console him saying, "Maybe this situation has happened for a reason. A reason that will unfold later."

In 1985, my grandmother passed away. She was seventy-one years old. Her death was a huge blow to Krishnamacharya. For many weeks after she died, he had a difficult time accepting that she was gone. There is a saying that behind every great man, there is a greater woman. Namagiriamma was Krishnamacharya's dedicated partner in life and in his mission to preserve and spread the teachings of yoga. Though she was a very quiet person, her support of Krishnamacharya was always unquestionable.

Krishnamacharya began to prepare for his own transition into the next world. He had presided over the revival of yoga in his own country and helped to spread its teachings and practice to countries around the world. Thanks to his students and to their students, people from all parts of the globe were embracing the discipline of yoga.

Krishnamacharya was especially pleased with the work of one student, his own son Desikachar. Desikachar had studied with Krishnamacharya nearly three decades, longer than any other student. Krishnamacharya saw in him a teacher who understood the potential of yoga and the richness and depth of its teachings, someone who would take yoga beyond *asana* practice and the obsession with physical performance found in too many yoga circles today. Desikachar would carry his legacy into the future, not only as his son, but also as his closest, longest-standing student. Desikachar had turned out to be a true *antevasin*—a student who stays until the end.

Krishnamacharya spent many hours during those last few years of his life teaching Desikachar from the texts he valued most highly and considered the most useful to society. These included the *Yoga Sutra*, *Bhagavad Gita*, *Hatha Yoga Pradipika*, *Yoga Yajnavalkya*, *Yoga Rahasya*, *Gheranda Samhita*, *Siva Samhita*, *Caraka Samhita*, *Samkhya Karika*, *Rahasya Traya Sara*, *Ramayana*, *Mahabharata*, *Paniniya Siksa*, the most important *Upanishads*, and many more. He also instructed Desikachar in *Ayurveda*, Yoga Therapy, basics of astrology, and the most important meditation practices.

All of the great yoga masters have elaborated on the teachings of Patanjali, providing their own interpretations and explanations of the *sutras*. Desikachar had been trying to get Krishnamacharya to write a commentary on the *Yoga Sutra* for years, and finally, he agreed. Because he was quite old and could not write easily for long periods of time, he chose to dictate the entire book to Desikachar, passing it on orally and in Sanskrit language, as such teachings have been passed on for thousands of years.

This dictation process became another lesson for Desikachar. He recalled, "I would be surprised at how he would exactly remember what he had dictated the day before. He would close his eyes and begin dictating in Sanskrit and sometimes when he would make references to a different text, he would even quote the exact chapter and verse number of the quotation. Being curious, I would go later to check if it matched with the exact chapter and number, and he was never wrong. Every time he would quote perfectly. I am amazed that one man could do and be so much."

Krishnamacharya's commentary on the *Sutras*, *Yogavalli*, presents the teachings of Patanjali as Krishnamacharya understood them. His interpretations are rich and insightful, and they bring the *Sutras* to life in a way that makes them more understandable to the reader.

For example, Krishnamacharya uses a simple analogy from everyday life to help us understand the concept of yoga as a *samskara* or a preparation process. "The mind," he says, "is like a vessel used for cooking. I have just used the vessel to make some soup. However, I want to boil milk with the same vessel. What

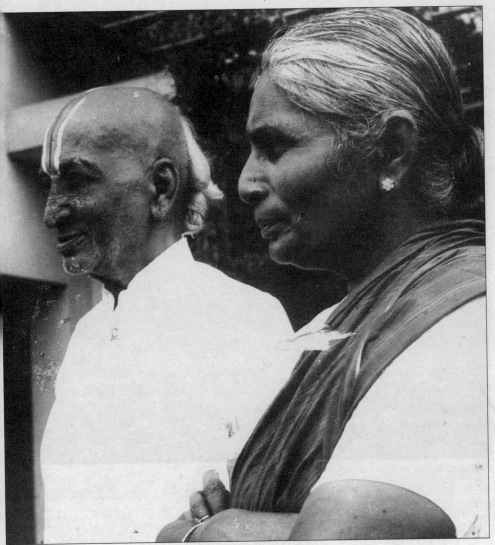

Krishnamacharya with Namagiriamma—one of the strongest pillars of his life.

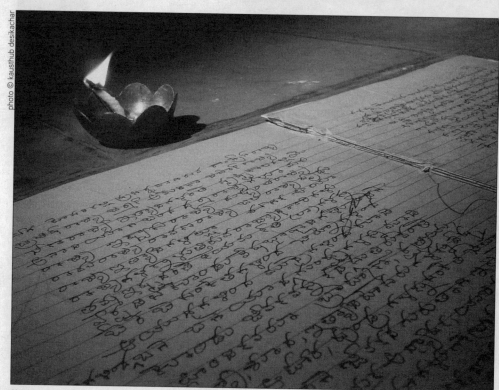

Krishnamacharya's writings, in his own hand.

do I do? I clean the vessel so that it becomes ready for boiling milk. It's the same with yoga. Our mind is the vessel that is used for many purposes. It carries impressions from our past actions, and we do not want these impressions to affect our future actions. So we need to go through a preparation process that cleans the vessel and makes it fit for future action."

In *sutras* I.23 through I.29, Patanjali discusses meditation on God. Few masters have elaborated on this section in their commentaries, probably because they lived during a period of time when yoga and *Vedanta*, the religious tradition, were more connected. The ancient masters would have taken for granted that people already knew how to meditate on God, so they would not have felt a need to comment on this section. However, today, when people from many different cultures, traditions, and belief systems practice yoga, this assumption can no longer be made. Krishnamacharya recognized this, and so he set down clear guidelines for meditating on God that can be followed by anyone, no matter what their religious background. This is what makes *Yogavalli* one of Krishnamacharya's most extraordinary gifts to us.

Once *Yogavalli* was finished, Krishnamacharya began to dictate another commentary to Desikachar, this one on the *Vedanta Sutra*. *Vedanta Sutra* is the fundamental text for every religious school in India. It was composed by a great saint, Veda Vyasa, and is the sixth Indian *Darsana*, or philosophy. The focus of *Vedanta Sutra* is the understanding and realization of God, or *Brahma*, who is presented as a Supreme Being devoid of form, name, and nature. Also called the *Brahma Sutra*, this text has been interpreted by various masters over the ages, which resulted in the splintering of *Vedanta* into many different, often conflicting schools.

Krishnamacharya's family followed the *Sri Vaisnava* tradition that evolved out of the *Vedanta* teachings of Nathamuni, Yamunacarya, Ramanuja, and Vedanta Desikacarya. It is likely that Krishnamacharya felt it was his duty as a lineage holder to write a commentary on the *Vedanta Sutra*, especially since he had refused the call to preside as Pontiff at the Math School more than once.

Krishnamacharya titled his finished work, *Cit Acit Tattva Mimamsa*. Literally translated, this means "An Inquiry into *Cit*, *Acit*, and *Tattva*." *Cit* refers to the consciousness that exists in all beings, *Acit* refers to matter that supports the consciousness, which includes our body, mind, senses, etc., and *Tattva* refers to that source of all of these, which we may call God. *Mimamsa* means an inquiry or a study.

Krishnamacharya produced these two masterpieces, *Yogavalli* and *Cit Acit Tattva Mimamsa*, during the last years of his long and glorious life. Maybe this was the reason Namagiriamma spoke of when she would console him after he broke his hip and lost some of his personal independence. Many people choose to rest or even withdraw from the world in their final years, particularly when they become frail, but Krishnamacharya chose to continue on the path appointed to him by his teacher so many years before, thanks to the inspiration of his wife.

Krishnamacharya also began teaching *Vedic* chanting to women. This was extremely controversial at the time, because, traditionally, *Vedic* chanting was taught only to men. Krishnamacharya himself when he was much younger had written an essay defending the prohibition against woman learning to chant. But as he matured, his opinions changed.

Mala Srivatsan, a student of Krishnamacharya's, was one of the first women to have the honor of learning the art of Vedic chanting from him. It was also a personal triumph for Mala to be chanting with her teacher. She first sought out Krishnamacharya years before to gain relief from an asthma condition, and she would never have imagined then that, one day, she would be capable of chanting.

Soon, Krishnamacharya began teaching chanting to other women, and this created an uproar in the community. Many people thought Krishnamacharya had lost his mind, or at the very least, that age had impaired his judgement. Krishnamacharya answered his critics with quotations from the ancient texts, including the *Ramayana* and *Yoga Yajnavalkya Samhita*, in which women are described as chanting the *Vedas*. He even invited authorities on the topic to debate him and prove him wrong, but none came forward. He continued teaching women to chant, and no one challenged him again.

Krishnamacharya would later comment, "In these times when those who are supposed to learn chanting (men) are not interested in learning it, we have to teach it to anyone who is willing to learn. Otherwise, this tradition will die." Now, hundreds of women are practicing and learning *Vedic* chanting and reaping its benefits. In fact, our *Vedic* Chanting Department at the KYM is run entirely by female teachers.

It was 1988. Krishnamacharya's hundredth birthday was approaching, and his students wanted to put together a special celebration. Ever the humble teacher, Krishnamacharya refused.

Hoping to get his father to change his mind, Desikachar decided to remind Krishnamacharya of an incident that had taken place years ago when Krishnamacharya was teaching at the *Yoga Shala* and working closely with the King of Mysore.

The King wanted to honor the Pontiff of the Parakala Math with an eightieth birthday celebration, but the Pontiff refused to allow any kind of party to be planned for this day. The King called on Krishnamacharya to help him convince the Pontiff to allow the celebration.

The Pontiff argued that it would be like "blowing your own horn" if he approved such a gathering, and hence, an act of ego. Krishnamacharya assured him that this was not the case; rather, the celebration was an act of gratitude performed by the students on his behalf. Krishnamacharya's reasoning changed the Pontiff's mind, and he agreed to take part in the celebration.

When Desikachar reminded him of this story, Krishnamacharya agreed to take part in the celebration on one condition: that it be an offering to God, and not to him. His students happily accepted these terms.

However, this celebration would have its own share of dramas. In the midst of the preparations, our family

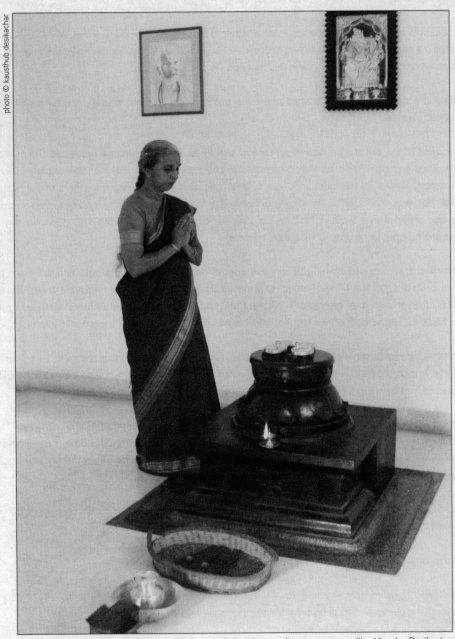

Ever since Krishnamacharya opened the doors of chanting to all, many women like Menaka Desikachar (seen here practicing at the *Sannidhi*) have become adepts in this ancient art.

doctor, who was attending to my grandfather's needs at that time, told my father, "Stop the preparations for the celebrations. I don't think he will live that long."

Everyone was confused. No one could decide whether to proceed with the plans or not. When Desikachar reported the doctor's words to his father, Krishnamacharya replied sternly, "I know my *prana*. I have given my commitment that I will participate in this function. Go ahead, don't stop."

Desikachar accepted his teacher's word as the final one on this matter and preparations for the birthday festivities resumed.

Every detail of the celebration was taken care of exactly as Krishnamacharya requested. There were one hundred and eight *Vedic* scholars assembled to chant the *Vedas, Ramayana, Mahabharata, Srimad Bhagavatam*, as well as the most important poems composed by *Sri Vaisnava* teachers of the past. A special ritual was conducted as an offering to God and to protect and serve society. The Governor of the State also presided over a public function honoring the centenarian on November 14th 1988, the day he turned one hundred (according to the Indian calendar).

Krishnamacharya received many gifts on this special occasion, including a gold pendant from the *Sankaracarya* of Kanci Math. This gift touched Krishnamacharya very much. The men were great admirers of each other, though they belonged to different philosophical schools (*Sankaracarya* belonged to the *Saiva* tradition). But respect draws respect, and this was the case with these two great masters.

Krishnamacharya's students also asked their teacher for a gift, his own *padukas* (sandals). Later, during the same year on the last day of *Navaratri* (a very auspicious day in India), Krishnamacharya symbolically transferred his powers to the *padukas* and asked his students to protect them.

In January 1989, Krishnamacharya summoned Desikachar to his side and handed him an old book. "This is a copy of the *Ramayana*," he told his son. "Before my father died, he gave me this book and said 'this is the only wealth you must have.' And this book has ever since been dear to me all my life. My only wealth has been the message of this book, and I now want to give this to you."

Desikachar was honored and overwhelmed to receive this book from his father, but his pleasure at the gift was overshadowed by his sense that Krishnamacharya's life was drawing to an end.

But Krishnamacharya had more than a gift for Desikachar, he had a request.

"My last wish," Krishnamacharya told him, "is also that you remain in Madras and not move to Mysore. I want you here, because good people like MV Murugappan live here."

Such was Krishnamacharya's fondness for Chennai and its residents, especially for MV Murugappan and his family.

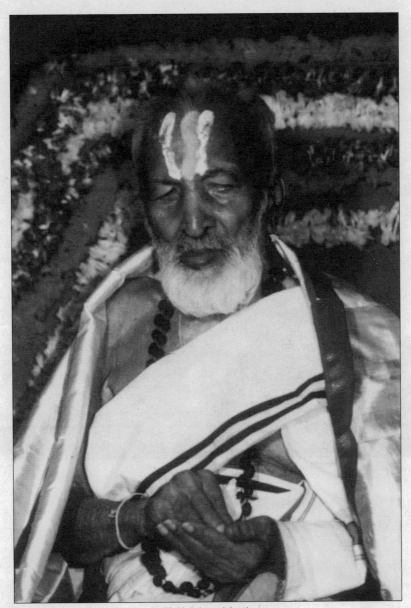

Krishnamacharya during the hundredth birthday celebrations.

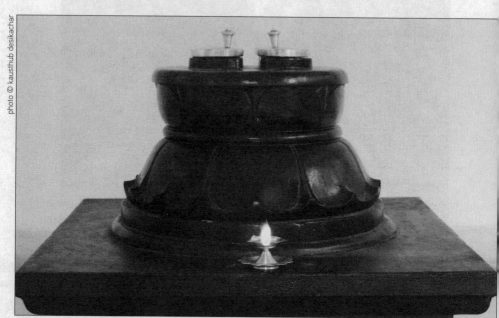

photo © kausthub desikachar

The *padukas* (sandals) of T Krishnamacharya, in the *Sannidhi*.

Desikachar had spent more than five years building a home in Mysore, intending to move the family there after his father died, but he immediately called a friend in Mysore and told him to sell the house. When his friend expressed disbelief, Desikachar replied simply, "It is my father's last wish that I remain here in Madras, so I am not moving to Mysore."

On February 28, 1989, at around 4:00 p.m., Krishnamacharya breathed for one last time. A glorious life ended. But Krishnamacharya left behind a rich legacy that will keep his spirit alive for many years to come. His life ended in 1989, but his mission is carried on through the work of his students and in the teachings.

"When I was studying all these [subjects] with my father," my father told me during one of our discussions about my grandfather, "many times I would wonder if I would ever need all these teachings. I was doing well within the limited tools that he had taught me. However, I see the value for all these teachings now, after his death. When I have doubts and situations when I can't consult him like I would do before, almost always I find the answers in the teachings he has shared with me. I feel very fortunate for being blessed in this manner."

The *padukas* Krishnamacharya gave to his students, the symbol of a teacher's wisdom and immense spirit, rest today in a place we call *Sannidhi* and continue to serve as a great source of inspiration and healing.

Krishnamacharya's way of teaching yoga encompassed every aspect of human life. Through his own life's example, as well as his teaching, he revived the message of the ancient masters that yoga is a holistic healing system that improves the way we live. For Krishnamacharya, Patanjali was "*the yogi*," and Patanjali's yoga was "**the yoga**." If we had to sum up the work of Krishnamacharya in one line, I would say that he revived "**the yoga of *the yogi*.**"

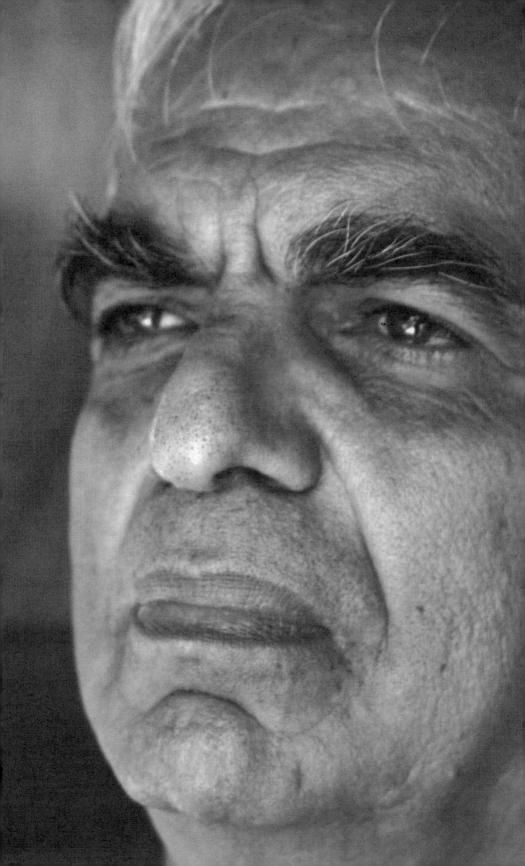

Chapter Ten

The Son Is Shining
carrying the legacy into the future

the sun does not set permanently,
it merely sets only to arise again.

When my father bought our house in the early 1970s, there was a drumstick tree on the north-east side of the property. In India, there is an old superstition that says if there is a drumstick tree on the land, a ghost haunts that place. This tends to discourage potential buyers.

But when my father showed the land to my grandfather and mentioned this tree, my grandfather said, "Ghost!!! No ghost will harm us. If there is indeed any ghost, it will only protect us, as we are followers of Lord *Narayana*. We are moving into this house. Buy it." Never one to question my grandfather, my father bought the house, and we moved in.

It is fascinating for me to think about this now. The north-east side of our property is where the *Sannidhi* is located. It is a simple building. There is a neat verandah at the entrance and a square sanctum. The building is painted white, with a traditional brick tile roof topped by a metallic crown. Six large windows look out onto gardens, and natural light brightens the single room inside. Directly opposite the entrance to the *Sannidhi* at the other end of the garden is a statue of Patanjali, the great sage, seated in peaceful meditation. Between the *Sannidhi* and Patanjali there is a small pond. Lotus and lily weeds float on the clear water and below them, you can catch a glimpse of swimming fish. At each corner of the pond, there is a statue of a *yogi*, and each *yogi* is performing a different yoga pose. These four statues represent the four students of Patanjali, for whom, according to legend, each chapter of the *Yoga Sutra* was written.

The word *Sannidhi* means, literally, "good space" or "appropriate space." What better place to lay Krishnamacharya's sandals to rest, than in this good space where he spent the last few years of his life? It is almost as if Krishnamacharya is living there still. When I am inside the *Sannidhi*, I feel the same feelings my grandfather inspired in me when he was alive: serenity, awe, fear, and most importantly, faith. My grandfather's words about this good space were prophetic; whatever ghost wanders this place now will surely protect us.

There is a *sutra* in Patanjali's *Yoga Sutra* that elucidates the concept of *Sannidhi*.

> **ahimsa pratisthayam tat sannidhau vairatyagah | Yoga Sutra II. 35**
>
> *one who has firmly established himself in ahimsa, in his mere presence, all evil will be cast away*

In other words, in the presence (in the *sannidhi*) of those who have always stood for *ahimsa* (non-violence), evil fades away and only good remains.

Krishnamacharya lived a life devoted to service. He healed thousands of people directly, and he healed thousands more through the efforts of the students he trained. These students then went on to train others, multiplying the reach of his personal wisdom. He worked all of his life to alleviate suffering and never caused harm. This is why people feel only good when they enter the *Sannidhi*. They experience the same feelings of compassion, healing, and friendship in the *Sannidhi* that Krishnamacharya inspired in us when he was alive.

Recently, my father was called in to settle a dispute between two brothers. The brothers were unwilling to compromise with each other in any way, and my father soon found himself running out of solutions. Finally, he decided to bring the brothers together in the *Sannidhi*. They sat face-to-face while he chanted one of his favorite passages from one of our *Upanisads*, the *Narayana Upanisad*.

By the end of the chanting, the two brothers were in tears and embracing one another. My father knew at that moment that he did not need to worry about finding a solution anymore, the dispute had been resolved.

More recently, my father and I again sought refuge in the *Sannidhi*. My student Karina, who is in her early forties, was trying to have a child, without success. Although the situation was looking hopeless, she did not want to give up on her desire to be a mother and raise a family with her husband. I decided to take her to see my father and ask him to bless her.

My father had known Karina for some time, and he told me to bring her to the *Sannidhi*, explaining that we should take blessings from Krishnamacharya himself. In the *Sannidhi*, he and my mother, Menaka, chanted for Karina. At the end of the chanting, my father gave Karina a bangle and asked her to wear it as a reminder that she had been blessed at the *Sannidhi*. In India, it is tradition to offer such symbols as a reminder of having visited a special place for a special reason.

This meeting at the *Sannidhi* took place in November 2003. While I was traveling in New Zealand in January 2004, I got a call from Karina in the middle of the night.

"Are you pregnant?" I asked her. I was completely convinced that this was the reason she was calling.

"No, I am not," she said. "I am calling because I have a question to ask you about my nose. It is quite cold here in Sweden, and my nose has become numb."

I helped Karina with this problem, and then I went back to sleep and had a strange dream. In the dream, I saw Karina with a boy seated on her lap. She and the boy were alone in a room. Soon, the boy got up and left the room, and a little girl came in and sat on Karina's lap and stayed there.

When I woke up, I called my father and told him about the dream and about Karina's phone call during the night. He told me, "Probably you are expecting her to be pregnant, and this is why such an expression came in your dream."

Three weeks later, I was in Melbourne teaching at a center run by my friend Barbara, who was also

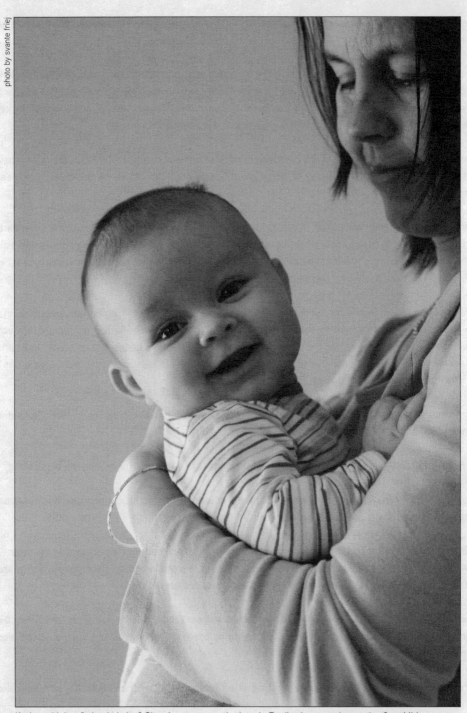

Karina with her "miracle baby." She always wears the bangle Desikachar gave her at the *Sannidhi*.

Karina's first yoga teacher. Barbara and I were sitting at a café drinking coffee, when we received a phone call. It was Karina.

I was much more cautious this time, asking her only, "How is your nose?"

"Kausthub," she said excitedly, "how did you know that I was pregnant when I called you three weeks ago? I have just returned from the doctor's office, and they have confirmed that I am three weeks pregnant."

I told Karina about my dream, thinking to myself: the magic of Krishnamacharya continues. When Hilma was born in September 2004, Karina called her "the miracle baby." Karina has never met my grandfather, yet he blessed her through my father, through the *Sannidhi*.

The moment I knew that her child, Hilma, was a girl, I knew that the little boy who had climbed down from Karina's lap in my dream was the child she had miscarried earlier. She told me later that she had always thought herself to be the mother of a little girl.

Some would dismiss all of this as coincidence. Others would contend that it was the brothers' faith and Karina's faith in Desikachar that made the difference, and no one would argue with that point.

But if you were to ask Desikachar himself, he would say, "It's because of my teacher, what he taught me, and my own faith in him."

Faith is at the heart of yoga. Desikachar will only take those who show absolute faith into the *Sannidhi*. For him, it is a place of healing, devotion, and spiritual transformation.

"[The *Sannidhi*] is not a temple or some place of worship for anyone to come and visit. Nor is it a tourist destination. It is a sanctuary of faith that is only special to those who value it," he always says.

After Krishnamacharya's death, the fate of his teachings was not clear to everyone. Some even thought that once he died, his whole teaching would die with him. If this had happened, Krishnamacharya would never have been a great master, because every great master in the past has ensured the continuity of the tradition through what is called the *guru parampara*.

Guru parampara is an Indian concept having to do with the transfer of knowledge and tradition. Beginning with the very first teacher, the teachings are handed down from one generation to the next through this *parampara*, or lineage. In each generation, a chosen student becomes the *pratinidhi* (torch bearer) of the teacher and the teachings and carries the legacy of the master into the future.

Krishnamacharya considered himself to be merely a *pratinidhi* in this long lineage of teachers. This is why he always said that the teachings were not his own, but belonged to the masters who preceded him.

161

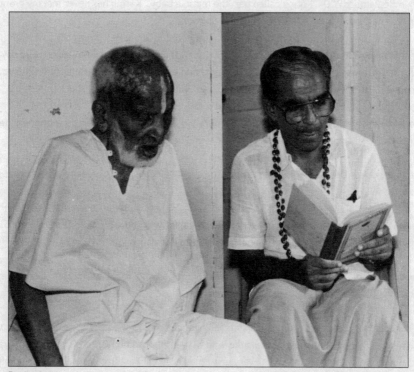

Desikachar learning some of the finer aspects of the *Upanisads* from Krishnamacharya.

"You are like a thief," he would say, "if you consider that these teachings belong to you. Even Patanjali did not claim [them] as his own. So how can we claim [them] as ours? [The teachings] only belong to the *parampara*, the *parampara* that was started by the first teacher ever."

In a world in which everyone is keen on patenting and brand-naming everything, including yoga, this way of thinking is rare and serves as an example of the true spirit of yoga.

Krishnamacharya had many students, but none were as close to him as his son Desikachar. This closeness did not arise only out of their father-son relationship, because Krishnamacharya loved all of his children, but he did not establish this particular kind of relationship with them. Desikachar was so close with Krishnamacharya, because he studied with his teacher longer than any other student. From the moment he became a student of his father, there was no looking back for Desikachar. His passion for yoga was ignited, and he never gave it up. Over the course of a long, intense education, Krishnamacharya taught Desikachar nearly all that was useful for the continuation of his teaching, because Desikachar was Krishnamacharya's *pratinidhi*. And as *pratinidhi*, he would fulfill his duty to his teacher and to the teachings.

Wherever I travel in the world, people come up and ask me why my father's teachings are so different from other students of Krishnamacharya, especially BKS Iyengar or Pattabhi Jois. My reply is always the same: Desikachar was a student of Krishnamacharya longer than anyone else. The others were his students for a much shorter time.

Also, BKS Iyengar and Pattabhi Jois were teenagers when they first began working with Krishnamacharya, so Krishnamacharya taught them *asana*-based teachings, the yoga most appropriate for this stage of their lives. The focus of their yoga practice was dynamic postures done as a *vinyasa*, which respected their younger stage of life.

For this reason, Iyengar's and Jois's teaching today is dominated by *asanas*. And if you look at it carefully, their *asana*-based teaching is superior to the teaching offered in traditions not linked with Krishnamacharya, because of the solid training they received from Krishnamacharya when they were young men.

Desikachar's experience with Krishnamacharya was quite different. He began teaching yoga as a young man in the 1960s, but he remained a student of his teacher until 1989, when he himself was in his fifties. Surely, what was applicable to him as a young man was quite different from what he needed in his forties and fifties. Working with his teacher throughout this thirty-year period, from boyhood to adulthood, allowed him to learn and experience a wide range of practices appropriate to each stage of life.

Desikachar was also fortunate enough to live with his teacher. He had the opportunity to refine his teaching, to model it on Krishnamacharya's example to a degree not possible for someone who did not live in such close proximity to him. This is why Desikachar's teaching resembles his father's. It is also why

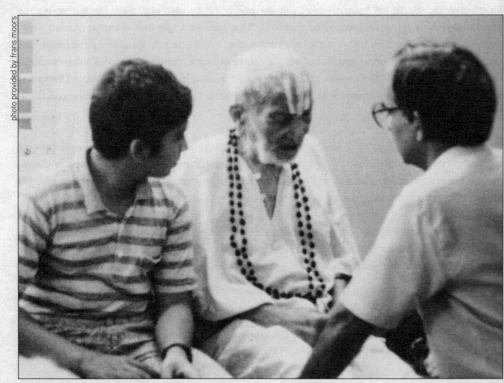

Three generations: Krishnamacharya, flanked by Desikachar and Kausthub (on his right).

Desikachar does not rely solely on *asanas* or *pranayama*, but like his father, he mastered the entire range of tools that yoga has to offer, and he utilizes them all, as appropriate, in his teaching.

"Teach what is appropriate to the student, and not what is appropriate to us." This is the truth at the heart of Krishnamacharya's teaching, and Desikachar honors this truth.

For example, when Desikachar is with a youngster who is interested in promoting strength and flexibility, he teaches dynamic sequences or *vinyasa krama*. If he is working with a pregnant lady, he teaches her with gentle *asanas* and *pranayama* to help her find peace of mind, as well as flexibility around the pelvis to aid her in giving birth. An elderly gentleman seeking to meditate on God, usually receives a meditative practice that revolves around his personal belief system.

In gratitude to his father for the teachings he received from him, Desikachar founded the Krishnamacharya Yoga Mandiram in 1976. This center is a nonprofit institution that continues to focus on sharing the wealth of Krishnamacharya's work through teaching, Yoga Therapy, and programs that bring yoga to the socially and economically challenged. The KYM also promotes Krishnamacharya's teachings through publications and yoga education. Today, the center attracts serious *yogis* who want to dive more deeply into the ocean of yoga.

Desikachar is to Krishnamacharya what Madhurakavi was to Nammalvar. It was Madhurakavi who made the world take notice of Nammalvar, a humble but great *yogi*. Similarly, even though many people in India and the world knew of Krishnamacharya and deeply respected his work, it is Desikachar who shined the light on the complete spectrum of his father's work after his death, bringing it to the attention of an even wider audience. It was to Desikachar that Krishnamacharya first spoke about *Yoga Rahasya*, to Desikachar that he dictated his commentaries on the *Yoga Sutra* and *Vedanta Sutra*, and to Desikachar that Krishnamacharya taught so many precious teachings.

And then at the end of his life, Krishnamacharya passed on his copy of the *Ramayana*, given to him by his own father years before, to his son Desikachar.

Today, Desikachar continues his mission of preserving his father's legacy and sharing it with others. Though retired from his administrative work at the KYM, he is still very active in teaching and training the center's teachers. He also spends a great deal of time translating and organizing his father's teachings and traveling around the world bringing the message of the ancient tradition of yoga to a new generation. Through him, the *parampara* continues into the twenty-first century.

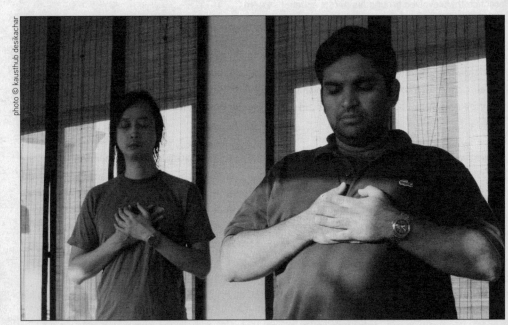

Kausthub Desikachar leading a student through an early morning meditation to the sun.

Epilogue

As I sat in my beautiful, comfortable room in a hotel in New York, one of two thousand students and teachers gathered in this luxurious space to participate in a yoga conference, I couldn't help thinking that the world of yoga has changed dramatically in the last hundred years.

In the early part of the twentieth century, yoga was practiced by very few people, most of them Indian ascetics living in caves, mountains, or forests. Their small community of *yogis* and yoga students commonly practiced only twenty to thirty postures (difficult for us to imagine today), even though the ancient texts indicated that there were thousands.

Then Krishnamacharya returned from Mt. Kailash in the early 1930s after training with his teacher for almost eight years. He brought with him the knowledge of hundreds of yoga postures, as well as a method of teaching that would help to revive the yoga tradition in India and carry it beyond India's borders to the rest of the world.

Today, yoga is practiced by people in every corner of the world, from every kind of background. School children and children with special needs, the elderly, stressed executives, prisoners, sick people, healthy people, addicts in recovery, expectant mothers, the rich and the poor, Christians, Muslims, Hindus, Jews, Buddhists, etc. They are all practicing yoga, reaping its benefits in one form or another. This would have been inconceivable to a *yogi* or to any Indian in the early twentieth century.

Tirumalai Krishnamacharya deserves most of the credit for this revolutionary revival. "Teach yoga," his teacher told him. That was his mission. His *Guru Daksina*. Simple, yet, at a time when yoga was on the verge of becoming just an interesting footnote in Indian cultural history, a monumental undertaking for one man.

Krishnamacharya succeeded. And along the way, he remained the same man, selfless and humble. He never sought fame or benefit for himself. Despite his accomplishments, despite the adulation and respect of his community, he died a simple man in a humble home. He had no need for more. He had done what he set out to do with his life.

Trying to contain this colossal life in one small book is an impossible task. Beyond the obvious challenges, there are simply many aspects of his life we will never know anything about. In those times, people did not keep official records or journals, relying on memory instead. And though Desikachar and the other students often urged Krishnamacharya to share more about his life, he would begin to oblige them and then suddenly stop in the middle and say, "If I continue it's like I am blowing my own trumpet." In the end, what we know of him is like one leaf, compared to the banyan tree of what we do not know.

What I can offer from my own experience are memories of a family man, a husband who loved to spend time with his wife, a father and grandfather who loved his children and grandchildren. He was well past sixty when the *Yoga Shala* at Mysore palace closed, but he began his professional life all over again, not only so that he could carry on his mission, but also to provide for his family and make sure his children received the best education available. When grandchildren came along, he doted on every single one of them. He spent enormous amounts of time playing with us, telling us stories, and even taking us with him on his visits to the market where he would pick his own fruits and purchase ingredients for the *Ayurvedic* medications he prepared for his students.

While doing research for this book project, I went to the fruit shop my grandfather used to frequent. After I had chosen some fruits to buy, I engaged the seller in a conversation, hoping to turn up some gem of information. The middle-aged man helping me did not seem to know much, but the older man sitting behind the cash register, presumably the owner of the shop, asked me, "Are you the grandson of the old yoga man?"

My eyes gleamed. I said, "Yes, of course. Do you remember him?"

The old man called me over to his side and began to speak about Krishnamacharya with great respect. I asked him if he had learned anything from this "old yoga man."

"Commitment," the elder gentleman replied immediately. "He could have gone and bought his fruits from any one of the many shops on the street. We all sell the same fruits and prices are the same. Sometimes the prices are even cheaper from the neighbor's store. But he would never go anywhere else. He would choose one store—ours. This taught me about commitment. This is why I still remember him."

Only now, more than twenty years after his death, has the wider yoga community begun to take notice of Krishnamacharya and understand the richness of his legacy. Not only did he revive the practice of *asana* and *pranayama*, but also the ancient art of *Yoga Cikitsa*, or Yoga Therapy. *Yoga Rahasya*, the lost text that he recovered in a vision, is one of the few classical texts that discuss this art in any detail. Thanks to him, yoga is helping a wide variety of people today heal from injury and disease, while it enhances the quality of life for people at every level of health. Millions are looking to this ancient science as a valuable, holistic healing practice, and a complement to modern medicine.

Krishnamacharya also left us a wealth of knowledge that has yet to be shared, in the form of texts, translations, commentary, essays, and poetry, including *Yogavalli* and *Cit Acit Tattva Mimamsa*. Both of these texts will be published in English soon.

As a master of many philosophical traditions, Krishnamacharya understood that spirituality was different from religion. Religion was one kind of spiritual practice, but it was not the only one. By refusing to open the door to religious discrimination, he opened the door of yoga to everyone.

He wrote in one of the verses of his poem, *Yoganjalisaram*:

> *Your lord or mine, it does not matter,*
> *With a quiet mind, meditate with humility,*
> *The Lord, pleased [with your devotion] gives what you seek*
> *And happily will offer more.*

Perhaps his greatest gift as a teacher was this expansive spirit, the respect he showed for the individuality of each student. Yoga, for him, was a personal practice, an art for healing the individual person. This was why he was also a different teacher with each student; he became the teacher the student needed.

"Teach what is inside you," he always said, "Not as it applies to you. But as it applies to the other [who is receiving it]."

This way of thinking is the exact opposite of the attitude we typically encounter in today's world, obsessed as it is with classification, with fitting people into neat, impersonal categories. Into yoga classes where one size is expected to fit all.

Because much of the yoga community today focuses only on *asana* practice, and also because it was Krishnamacharya who shaped much of the *asana* tradition practiced today, some writers have tried to categorize him, calling him a **Hatha Yogi**. These writers err on two fronts. First, they do not understand the term *Hatha Yoga* correctly. Second, they do not know enough about Krishnamacharya to categorize him this way. If they had done their research, they would have realized that their assumptions are wrong.

The term *Hatha Yoga* appears in some of the classical yoga texts, especially *Hatha Yoga Pradipika, Siva Samhita*, and *Gheranda Samhita*, among others. The way the authors used this term in these texts is quite different from the way it is understood today. The word *Hatha* is derived from two syllables: *Ha* and *Tha. Ha* and *Tha* represent the dual energies that dominate our lives. Because *Ha* and *Tha* are not united (or balanced), we are affected by extremes, like excitement and suffering, heat and cold, etc.

According to the classical texts, when a person has reached the state of yoga, the dual energies meet and the person becomes balanced, calm, and serene. Such a *yogi* is no longer agitated or excited; he or she is basically unaffected by the extremes. This is what is called *Hatha Yoga*. It is the yoga (union) of *Ha* and *Tha*. Interestingly, many of the classical texts including *Hatha Yoga Pradipika*, mention that this merging of energies happens because of *pranayama*, not *asana*. Of course, the texts talk about *asanas* being used as preparation for *pranayama*, but *pranayama* is always referred to as the main tool for merging the two energies.

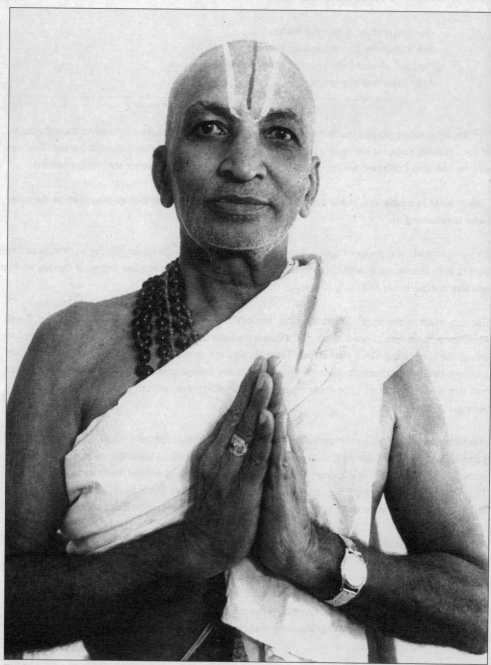

The Complete *yogi*, Krishnamacharya.

is probably the case that many of the writers and yoga practitioners who describe *asana*-oriented practices as *Hatha Yoga* do so, because one dictionary definition of the word *Hatha* is "forceful." Performing *asanas* with intensity or force then, some might conclude, must be *Hatha Yoga*.

This is not correct. *Asanas* themselves must never be done forcefully. When we see people forcing themselves into *asanas*, they are not calm or serene. They are often agitated, stressed, or aggressive. This is not consistent with the concept of *Hatha Yoga*.

t is my guess that this translation "forceful" refers to a practice that should be done with great willpower and strength, which is true for any yoga practice.

When we try to come up with a category to describe Krishnamacharya then, it is clearly a difficult task, because he was not one type of *yogi*. He is beyond these classifications which limit themselves to a single area of specialty, because he was a specialist in many areas. He was a **paripurna** *yogi*, a complete *yogi*. And his legacy to us is a complete yoga tradition, the depth and richness of which we are only beginning to understand.

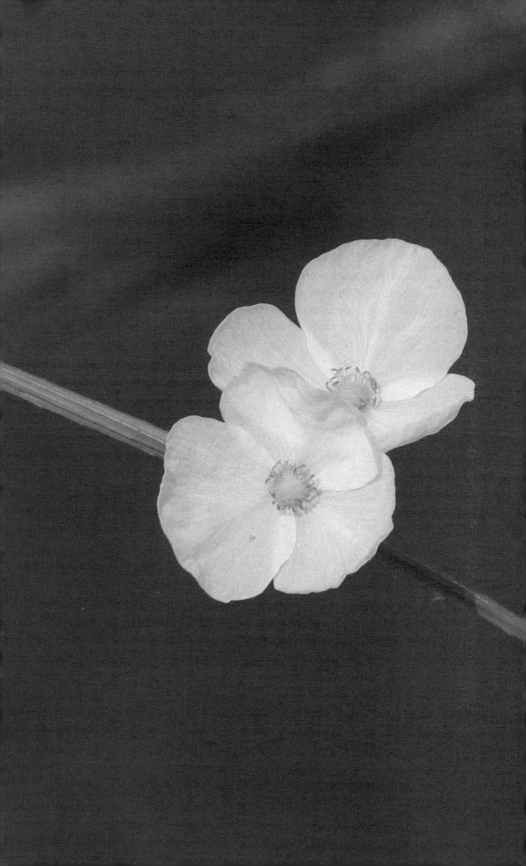

His Master's Voice
essays by students

In his lifetime, Krishnamacharya touched the lives of many people: students, friends, contemporaries, and his family and children. He left an impression on each heart. He taught lessons that altered lives and shared experiences that linger as fond memory.

In this section, we share a few essays written by people whose path in life intersected with Krishnamacharya's. Each essayist is different, and each path is different. Some contributors are yoga teachers, some are businessmen, some are housewives, and some are scientists. But what each writer shares with the other are memories of a great man. It becomes clear very quickly as you read through each story, what a multifaceted and inimitable man Krishnamacharya was, for though there are similarities among the writers' recollections, it seems that each one met a different person.

Perhaps, we can say that each student met the teacher they needed.

I want to thank each essayist, not only for taking the time to contribute to this book, but also for sharing the story of their personal odyssey with the grand master, Krishnamacharya.

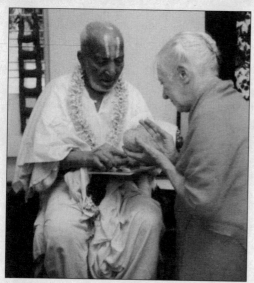

Indra Devi with her teacher, 1989.

Indra Devi

Indra Devi was the first foreign woman to study yoga with Krishnamacharya and one of his most famous students. She met her teacher in the 1930s in Mysore, and after studying with him for a few years, she went on to teach yoga to students all over the world. She returned to India in 1989 to meet with her teacher just before his hundredth birthday celebrations. Indra Devi settled in Argentina and lived there until her death at the ripe old age of 103. Her remarkable work continues to touch people's lives through Fundacion Indra Devi, based in Buenos Aires.

Author's Note: Indra Devi is the only person I was unable to interview. I received news of her death just after I sent her a letter about this book. Luckily, my friend, Larry Payne, had a video of her talking about Krishnamacharya during a commemorative event Larry organized in the 1980s. This essay is a summary of some of Indra Devi's commentary from that videotape.

It is a surprise to me to be here. Last Saturday, I was still in Argentina. It is to me [. . . at one stage] an honor and pleasure to be here and to honor my teacher, *Sri* Krishnamacharya.

Instead of just thanking this old, big human genius because he is one of the best teachers of yoga [and I always think that where Krishnamacharya's yoga teaching is concerned], I [wish] to say something about what it actually would have been [to be his student].

I saw him for [the] first time in Mysore. I think it was during *Dussera* (an Indian festival) and *Sri* [Krishnamacharya] was demonstrating to the guests of the *Maharaja*. He was doing yoga postures, and then at the end, he said, "If there are any doctors in the audience among the guests, [please] come and check—I am going to stop my heartbeat for several minutes."

And so *Sri* [Krishnamacharya] just took a breath and lay down on the floor. Very close to him was sitting a German doctor. He came back shaking his head and said, "I have pronounced him as dead." He had checked with a stethoscope and many doctors came [and checked] but they didn't have a thought. He said, "I don't understand it."

I asked him, "Doctor, you live in India. Wouldn't it be interesting for you to see what yoga can do?"

He said, "No."

I was ill for four years . . . I was cured by a medical student who knew how to apply the yoga that he had learnt. And then I showed him what I was doing and he said, "Be glad that something works. If you are doing the transmission of *prana*, it is from the hip to the toes, never back from the toes to the hip." And I was doing it up and down . . .

The end of the story was that I decided to come back to India and immediately start on the yoga training. And I remembered about Krishnamacharya. I started my yoga training in Bombay, at Kuvalayananda Ashram, under Swami Kuvalayananda. And then, I very much wanted to go to Mysore. [At that time, Krishnamacharya's school was in a wing of the Jaganmohan Palace and the *Maharaja* was a patron of the school]. I came first to present myself and ask him [to accept me as his student].

He had all the name, all the voice, all the influence in the school. He politely declined [my request], but since the *Maharaja* was a patron of the school, and I was the guest of the *Maharaja* and *Maharani* (queen), the *Maharaja* just asked him to accept me. And against his wish, he accepted me. His earnest desire was to see me behind the door as far as possible. So he put such a strong discipline on me that he knew very well I would not be able to follow it. "Wake up at four o'clock in the morning and before sunrise do this and that . . ." He wanted me to eat only sattvic food. You know—not even vegetables like carrots, potatoes, and radish that grow under the ground, only vegetables that ripen under the sun.

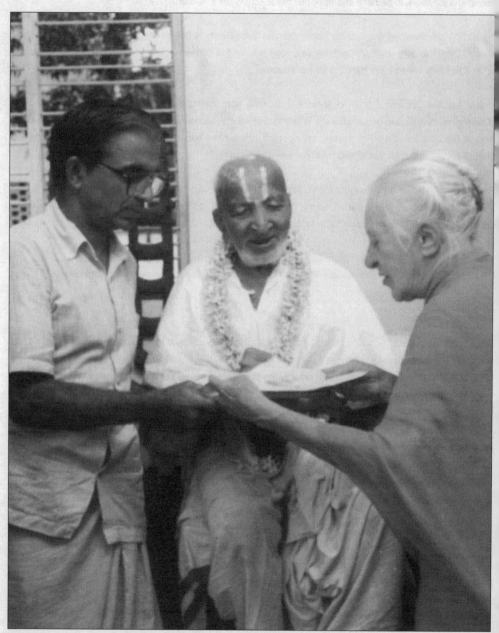
Indra Devi receiving blessings from her teacher. Desikachar looks on.

But the *Maharani* gave me a special cook, because she was a vegetarian and they were eating vegetables that grow in the sun. And when *Sri* [Krishnamacharya] finally saw that I meant it seriously, then he started taking interest in me and that was it.

My first husband was a diplomat in China, and I was staying in India. [I was going to China to join him] . . . And when I was leaving, Krishnamacharya told me, "Now that you will be in different countries . . . I want you to teach yoga." And I said, "Me? *Maf kariye* (please forgive me). I can't teach."

And I remember in one of the classes in the beginning, everybody was doing *Pascimatanasana* . . . forward bend . . . well, almost everybody . . . you know, feet stretched on the floor, and inhale—exhale you touch the toes. My hands were so far from the toes that I asked one of my co-students to push me from the back and *Sri* [Krishnamacharya] told me, "No, no, no! You can injure a muscle. You can do it by and by." And I remember I'm on the floor, looking up at him and saying, "In my next incarnation."

I never thought ever that I would be able to touch my toes.

End of the story, *Sri* [Krishnamacharya] insisted that I start teaching yoga. And he started giving me instructions and wanted me to write it down. In India you do not contradict your teacher. So I was writing down and thinking, "He is losing his time and mine."

On the boat from India to China, I knew that something totally changed my life. In the first place, I liked very much games, dancing, and you know rolling around. But for the first time in my life, even in the evening when I went up to the deck looking at the stars and meditating, I never danced. That was something nobody believed because dance [was something I loved].

I used to like going to cinemas and theatres, and I said I will continue to go to cinemas and theatres [even if I teach yoga]. I didn't think this would happen to me but I felt I had not to go. I lost interest in a lot of things including wearing jewels, wearing makeup . . .

It was my great luck and privilege to be able to spread yoga the way I was taught by *Sri* Krishnamacharya. And it was pure yoga. 🙶

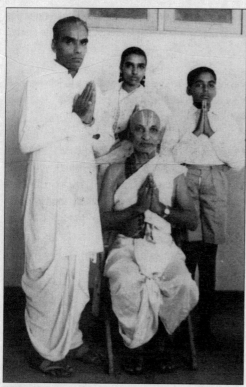

BKS Iyengar, Geetha Iyengar, and Prasanth Iyengar
with Krishnamacharya.

BKS Iyengar

BKS Iyengar, one of Krishnamacharya's most well-known students, met his teacher in the 1930s, when he became his brother-in-law. Mr. Iyengar studied under his teacher from 1934 to 1936, and then settled in Pune, India, where he continues to live and teach today. His work is known all over the world through the name of *Iyengar Yoga*, and his headquarters is the Ramamani Iyengar Memorial Yoga Institute. BKS Iyengar has authored many books, appeared in countless magazines, and *Time* magazine recently acknowledged him as one of the one hundred icons of the century.

Let me first salute my direct and revered *guru[ji]*, T Krishnamacharya, with respect and reverence, who happens to be my brother-in-law, my elder sister Namagiri's husband. Let me also invoke Lord Patanjali through prayers before I say something of my *guruji*, with all the humility at my command.

Firstly, it is very embarrassing and difficult to speak of my *guru[ji]*, who was a great man, a close relative, a versatile personality and at the same time a very hard taskmaster. It was no doubt a Herculean task to approach him. Secondly, my reverence for him as a great man may not allow me to do full justice. It is not easy for a pupil like me to talk of a master of such versatile character. Thirdly, I was hardly sixteen when I was his student. The time I lived and spent with my *guruji* was so short that it is not easy to sketch his lifestyle. My mind then was raw and childish. I do not think that I had developed much of an intelligence to study and understand him, nor was I in a position to taste the wisdom of his knowledge.

Guruji, no doubt, was a gifted and talented personality.

It is only possible to talk about such a person when the pupil is elevated to his master's level of intelligence.

I was a boy of seven-and-a-half years when he married my sister. He was thirty-three then and my sister was twelve. My first memory of him is the day of his wedding when he came with two elephants.

Guruji was a gifted man, with a very high intellectual calibre, powerful physical prowess and an unfaltering memory. I am sure he would have won the title of "Mr. Universe," if he had stood for such a contest. He was naturally gifted with a well-built body, proportionately muscular, expressing tremendous strength and vigor.

He was also a master of *Ayurveda*. He used to prepare *Ayurvedic* medicines and herbal oils such as "*lehyams*" (concoctions) and "*tailams*" (herbal oils) at home, which were very effective when used on his patients. But he never gave any clues as to how they were mixed and prepared.

Besides mastery in the fine art of music, he played *Karnatic* classical music on the *Veena* (a traditional Indian string instrument). *Guruji* was also a wonderful cook. He would cook only one or two dishes, but they used to be so tasty that I could never decide which one was the best. I used to call his preparations, *Madhupakam*—like honey.

He was a first-class gardener. He used to grow flowers and vegetables at his house in Mysore. He would sow any seed and by his magical touch, the plant would flourish.

Coming from an orthodox *Brahmin* family, he never used a charcoal fire for cooking, but would often cut wood with his own hands and used that as fuel. He used to enjoy cutting wood in the mornings from nine o'clock to eleven or twelve o'clock. He was precise in whatever work he did; whether cooking or cutting wood; singing *Vedic* hymns or playing the *Veena*. He would not tolerate any compromise or slackness with precision. He demanded the same from all of us. He was like a Zen master in the art of teaching.

You may not be knowing that after his marriage he got a job in a coffee plantation in the Hassan district of Karnataka. He used to dress differently, wearing half-pants and a half-sleeved shirt, socks and shoes, a hat on his head and a stick in his hand. It was unimaginable to see a man dressed in such a manner who had studied *Sat Darsanas* (the original six schools of Indian philosophy), with titles like *Samkhyayoga Sikhamani*, *Veda Kesari*, *Vedanta Vagisa*, *Nyayacarya*, *Mimamsaratna* and *Mimamsa-tirta*. He was an expert in *Vastu Sastra* (the science of scientific and aesthetic architecture) and *Jyotisa Sastra* (the science of Astrology).

In 1931, he left the plantation job and began giving lectures on philosophy. *Sri* Seshachar, a lawyer of Mysore, invited him to give a talk on the *Upanisads* in the town hall of Mysore. The event proved to be a turning point in his life. A hidden scholarly personality, in that garb of half-pants, half-sleeved shirt, hat, socks, and shoes, was unearthed. His discourse on the *Vedas*, *Upanisads* and Yoga attracted the elite of Mysore. The news of this scholar and his scholarly debate reached the ears of the *Maharaja* of Mysore, His Highness Sri Krishnaraja Wodeyar IV. The *Maharaja* was attracted by his knowledge and personality and became his student in order to understand the scriptures and yoga. Soon, he appointed him to teach *Mimamsa* and yoga in the Sanskrit *Pathashala* (school) run by the *Maharaja*.

My *guruji* was a strict teacher. His students and even the *pandits* found it difficult to answer a question paper prepared by him on *Mimamsa*. The students protested against him, and the *Maharaja* soon agreed to replace him from the Sanskrit *Pathashala* and started a *Yoga Shala* at the Jaganmohan Palace of Mysore as he never wanted to lose such a personality. With this offer of a *Yoga Shala*, he kept the option open that *Guruji* could go to the *Yoga Shala* whenever he wished and gave him the recognition of "*Asthana Vidvan*"—the intelligentsia of the palace.

The *Yoga Shala* was meant only for the members of the Royal Family. Outsiders were permitted on special requests. Therefore, it was a formidable task for an outsider to get entry into the *Yoga Shala*. *Guruji* used to have only a few select outsiders with him apart from the members of the Royal Family, and I was fortunate to be one of them.

The classes at the *Yoga Shala* were mainly devoted to teaching one to attain perfection in *asana*, or *asanas* for health. The classes were held only in the evenings between 5:00 p.m. and 7:00 p.m., while the morning classes between 9:00 a.m. and 10:30 a.m. were meant for ailing persons.

Guruji had a frightful personality. His back used to be straight even when he was aged. His eyes were so powerful that anyone would be afraid to look into his eyes. Nobody could cross this intellectual giant. The *pandits* and scholars were afraid of him. I have attended a few of his talks in the early days. As a young and highly educated person, he was intellectually intoxicated. Nobody could equal him in the art of discussion. He could create Sanskrit stanzas on the spot. He was a *kavi*—poet. To some extent, I feel that he did not get a proper channel to expose his abilities.

People were nervous of him. He was a fast walker. Nobody could keep pace with him. Nobody could match his speed. If he were walking along one side of the pavement, the elite of Mysore would cross over to the other side.

I don't know what *Guruji* saw in me. Perhaps he recognized that while I had no strength, I had guts. He ignited the courage in me. He introduced me to my "self" within. Or, perhaps, he discovered my inner potentials.

One thing that was certain about *Guruji* was that he would never go to see anyone, however great they may be. He commanded such a respect that such great personalities (criminal lawyer, *Sri* Srinivasa Iyengar from Madras and Swami Yogananda of [the] USA) had come to the *Yoga Shala* to see him.

Guruji, in those days, stressed on demonstrations. There were several incidents when *Guruji* not only demanded a demonstration, but also asked me to perform unknown and undone *asanas*. You may be surprised to know that almost all the difficult *asanas* such as *Vrscikasana* and *Adhomukha Vrksasana*, I learnt in public performances only. Such was the way and style of teaching of my *guru*[*ji*] that he would often ask his students to perform new and difficult *asanas* in public, and that, too, without any prior intimation or warning.

In 1935, Dr. Bruce, a cardiologist, and Dr. Morcault, a psychology professor, visited Mysore to study the changes and stopping of the heartbeats through yogic discipline. My *guruji* was very fond of castor oil. He used to drink it as though it was ghee. Until the end of the experiment, which was going on for four to five days, he had castor oil everyday. On the sixth day of the experiment, the machine stopped. It wouldn't show any beats. At first, the doctors thought that there was a power failure but saw that the light outside the testing room was working. Soon, they realized that he had really stopped his heartbeats.

In 1955, two doctors from [the] USA came to Lonavla. I was then based in Pune, teaching. These doctors were doing some research on *pranayama*. They asked me to come to Lonavla. They wanted to test whether the blood pressure increased during *Salamba Sirsasana*. They took the readings of those who were at Lonavla. However, my blood pressure did not rise. They were surprised and asked me about *pranayama* and the stopping of heartbeats. I asked them to visit my *guruji* who was an expert in *pranayama*. My *guruji* permitted them to take the test when he was practicing. They took the test and admitted that my *guruji* was the first one who did something in *pranayama*, where the recording showed that the heartbeats had slowed down.

Guruji came to Pune many a time. Whenever he came to Pune, he gave lectures and we gave demonstrations. As *guru* and *sisya*, we were always together mentally, if not physically. I never crossed my *guruji's* word in spite of a few quarrels with him and that, perhaps, protected me throughout my life.

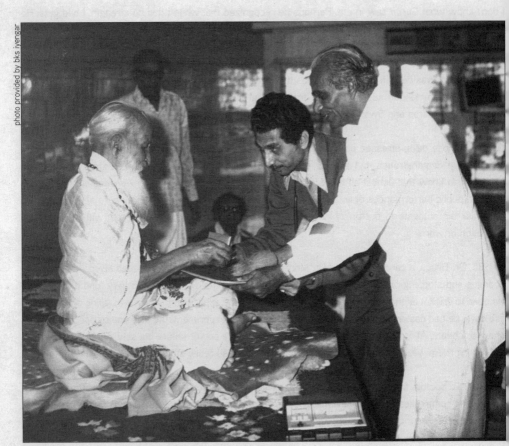

BKS Iyengar thanking Krishnamacharya for his visit to Pune, 1970s.

If he had been alive, he would have definitely read my commentary on the *Yoga Sutra*. I was a nonentity, but *Guruji* made me a hero. I was at the nadir in this subject. I climbed the tree of yoga step by step. Perhaps *Guruji's* eagle eyes made me think and rethink. Indirectly, he taught me to be totally aware. Today, I feel happy at heart and satisfied that I served my *guruji*.

I have lived with my *guruji*. I saw that he was not the same in Madras as he was in Mysore. He was as hot as fire in Mysore and as cool as water in Madras, a completely mellowed person. Yet, he was a top class teacher.

I must emphasize that the credit of success and popularity in yoga goes to his foremost students, including myself, who were not more than half a dozen in number. These students carried the message of yoga imparted by *Guruji*, with sincerity, honesty and dedication, and a note of thanks must go to them for keeping the fire of yoga alive even to this day.

The merit of the success of his pupils entirely belongs to *Guruji*, who has remained as a light to us all. Whatever we know about *Guruji* and his work is just a bit here and there. He was like an ocean. Everyone has learnt something from him. But what each has learnt is not complete. We all have to come together and put all his words and works together. Only then can we know how big and great he was.

I salute my *guruji* from the bottom of my heart. 🙶

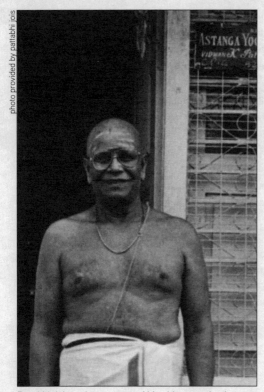

Pattabhi Jois at the entrance of his old yoga school.

Pattabhi Jois

Another famous student of Krishnamacharya, Pattabhi Jois, also met his teacher in the 1930s and was part of the famed *Yoga Shala* in Mysore. Today, Pattabhi Jois, known all over the world as the pioneer of what is now called *Astanga Vinyasa Yoga*, lived and taught out of his yoga school in Mysore up until his death in 2009. His grandson Sharath Rangaswamy, and his daughter, Saraswati Rangaswamy, continue to run the Sri K. Pattabhi Jois Ashtanga Yoga Institute in Mysore.

My father's father taught astrology. He was a *Vidvan* (professor). My father did not teach, but when people asked him questions, he would answer them. He was a good astrologer but I didn't take the time to learn it from him. He did teach me some astrology *slokas* every day and Sanskrit and the *Amarakosa* as well as *sabda* (phoenetics/syntax). After that, I would go to Hassan. I didn't go to the school in my village but to the one in Hassan, which was only five kilometres away. Everyday, I would walk to school in the morning and walk back in the evening. A lot of others came, too, including my friends. One day, when I had started studying at middle school, Krishnamacharya gave a lecture demonstration at the Jubilee Hall in Hassan. I didn't know who he was, but I went to see him anyway. My friend's sister told me that the man demonstrating was doing *asanas* perfectly, so I went along. I watched for an hour and I liked it completely. I thought to myself, "Tomorrow morning, I am going to his house and ask him to teach me," which I did. I told him my whole history. He said, "Tomorrow, you come."

So early next morning, I went to Hassan at 7:30 a.m. (school started at 10:30 a.m.), and went to the *guru*'s home, where he was teaching some students yoga practice, and I started that day. It was in 1927. I was a young man, so whatever *asana* I was told to do, I did quickly. My *guru* was very happy. After that, it was practice and more practice for two years. When my father finished my thread ceremony in 1930, I went to the Sanskrit college (the thread ceremony was required for entrance).

One day, after I had been at the college for a year, the principal put up a sign board asking if anyone knew wrestling, back bending, yoga, etc. If you did, he offered to let you do a presentation at the school's anniversary celebrations. I knew a few *asanas*. I didn't know the philosophy yet, but my *guru* was teaching it to me. The principal asked if I was doing yoga, and I said yes. So, on the anniversary day, I did yoga practice—this is *Pascimatanasana* . . . this is *Purvatanasana* . . . this is *Matsyasana*—I called out the *asanas* by name and then did them. It wasn't the full method by any means, but afterwards, he was very happy. The principal knew yoga, and he called me to his office the next day. He arranged for me to eat at the canteen and also gave me a scholarship.

Then, one or two years later, in 1932, a palace *Yoga Shala* was started by *Maharaja* Krishnaraja Wodeyar. In 1940, the *Maharaja* died. After him came his son and though he was also a good man, he wasn't interested in yoga. Some students at the time were saying that Krishnamacharya was a very hard man, that at the *Yoga Shala*, he wasn't taking complete care. But Krishnamacharya didn't care who you were. If an officer came, he wouldn't care. If that officer told him to do something, he would say, "Don't tell me what to do. I know very well. Go back to where you came from." A very tough man . . . So by 1952, he had gone to Madras. But, for about ten years before he left, I would go to his house every day at noon for the theory portion. He taught me and Mahadeva Bhatt the various methods of Therapy.

In 1936, a civil court judge, Gundu Rao, who lived near Bangalore, suffered paralysis. The *Maharaja* and my *guru* as well, told me to go and teach him. I went for about two months and taught him the complete Yoga Therapy. When I was done, he could walk and all his nervous problems were completely cured. After that, Krishnamacharya praised me.

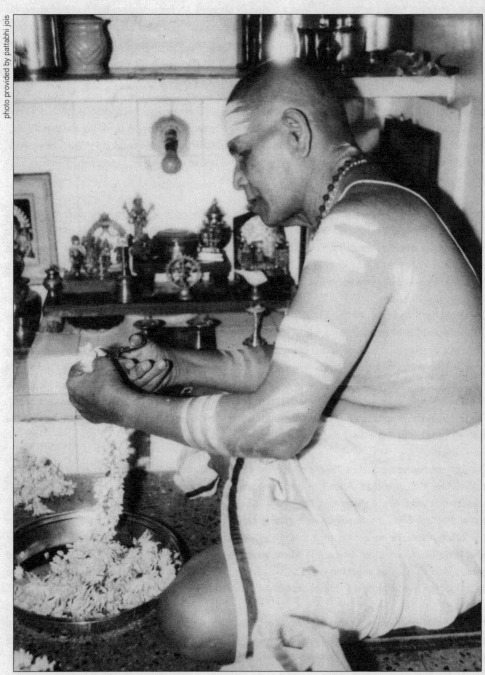

Pattabhi Jois preparing for a ritual.

traveled many times, teaching yoga. I also went to many places in India—Delhi, Calcutta, Bombay—researching and looking at all the yoga institutions. But, no. Only Krishnamacharya taught real yoga. He was a very great man, a very correct man. He was the only one in all of India. People today say they are doing yoga, but it is only a circus. There is no method, no breathing, no *vinyasa*, no *drsti* . . . only circus. In some places, the *guru* points to a picture and says, "do this." And then he leaves. This is not real teaching. Krishnamacharya was a fine man, a very good man, who taught very strictly and very precisely. He knew all the *sastras*. That is why he was able to teach yoga properly.

Once for my teaching certificate, Krishnamacharya said, "Here is a sick man, Cure him." Later he came and watched me and said, "Bad man! Is this teaching or hurting?" Then he corrected me. He was a good teacher. But afterwards, he would say, "Come to my house!" I would go and there would be lots of food. Krishnamacharya was teaching the real yoga, but this *Astanga Yoga* was very difficult. Teaching it is difficult, grasping it is also difficult. Without the right method, it is possible to get sick after starting. That is why you need a good teacher.

Krishnamacharya's eyes were very powerful. He only had to look at you for a second, and you'd be afraid. He spoke five languages perfectly—Hindi, Sanskrit, Telugu, Marati, and Kannada. Later, his English also improved.

In my entire life, I had only one *guru*. Two *gurus* are the cause of the death of the student. At the end of his life, Krishnamacharya and I were like father and son. My *guru*, Krishnamacharya, is always here, in my heart. 🙶🙶

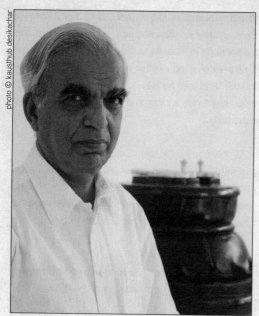

photo © kausthub desikachar

TKV Desikachar in front of his teacher's sandals.

TKV Desikachar

The youngest of Krishnamacharya's four most well-known students, Desikachar began to study yoga in the 1960s and continued learning with his teacher until 1989, the year Krishnamacharya died. Desikachar carries on his father's legacy through the Krishnamacharya Yoga Mandiram, where every aspect of Yoga and Krishnamacharya's teachings continues to be taught to new generations of students and teachers. Desikachar is the author and translator of many books, including *The Heart of Yoga*; *Health, Healing, and Beyond*; *What Are We Seeking?*; *In Search of Mind*; and *Reflections on Yoga Sutras*, among others.

Whenever we have to describe somebody else, it is normal, at least for me, that the presentation is what I see of the person. In this projection of Krishnamacharya, I must say that I have a sort of privilege because I lived with him. And I did not always agree with him. And therefore, it was possible to see certain things that I would not have if I had always been attached to him. It also happened that my interest in yoga was aroused only after I had completed my studies and was working as an engineer.

After I graduated in Engineering, I was working in Gujarat. I had just got a job in Delhi, and before I went there, I wanted to visit Madras to spend some time with my family. Then, we were staying in a very small apartment in a little lane of Gopalapuram, in Madras. My parents and my siblings stayed all together in that little place. While my father was an ardent practitioner and master of yoga, I had never got seriously involved in yoga.

One morning, as I sat reading the newspaper, a car stopped in front of my house and a foreign lady stepped out. She called out, "Professor" to my father, and then to my surprise she gave him a broad hug. I was completely taken aback that my father whom I had never even seen holding my mother, was allowing this lady, a foreigner at that, to hug him. When she left, I asked him about this incident. He told me that she was from New Zealand and had been suffering from severe insomnia. For the first time the previous night, she had slept without medication. She had now come to thank her teacher.

This incident had a very profound impact on me. What struck me was that this man, who had no exposure to Western systems of medicine, and who had no knowledge of modern science, had cured a foreigner who had access to the best medical facilities. I felt that I must learn more about this ancient discipline that my father practiced, and I requested him to teach me.

He said, "You will have your class at 3:30 a.m." My father would sleep in the kitchen, while the rest of us slept in one hall. I was ready the next morning at 3:30 a.m. My father began with a few verses from the *Hatha Yoga Pradipika*.

Then, I barely knew any Sanskrit and my voice was also very hoarse. These morning sessions were, therefore, quite a disturbance for my entire family, who were forced to wake up at that early hour. But, I knew that my father was testing my seriousness, and so I did not ask him to change the timing of my lessons.

Instead of going to Delhi, I decided to stay back in Chennai and become a student of my father. I took up a job at L&T in Chennai. It was all thanks to this one woman from New Zealand, that I got the urge to study yoga.

I was the last in my family to begin practicing yoga. When my father left for Madras in the '50s, I was in high school and cricket was a far more interesting proposition than yoga. I had been very keen on doing Engineering, but after I began learning yoga, I used my professional qualifications only as a means of income, for my heart was in yoga. In fact, my father had wanted me to take up the civil service examinations and was very disappointed that I did not become a gazetted officer.

A few months later, my boss at L&T asked me to stay back for a meeting after 5:15 p.m. As I had a ticket to a movie that evening, I lied and told my boss that I had to leave as I had a yoga class to teach. He permitted me to leave, but then added that he wanted me to teach him too the very next day.

First thing the next morning, my boss called to remind me that I had to teach him yoga that day. I had no choice but to teach him. And so I found that in a matter of a week, I had some fourteen students. And that is how I began my career as a yoga teacher.

When I began to study with him, my father was in his early seventies. I had heard that in his younger days, my father was a very strict and tough man. But I faced no such problems. He was always so kind to me in spite of the fact that I was not well-versed in philosophy, not very good in chanting, and not very flexible. My scientific education made me doubt his claim that he could stop his heartbeat at will. When he proved to me that he could do just that, then my trust in him became total. In all these ways, I consider myself one of his worst students, for so many others did his bidding unquestioningly and had such faith in his teachings.

When I was born, he was fifty years old. He had an immense educational background in everything except, perhaps, English. Initially, I found it hard to believe that he was so well-educated, but after having studied with him for about thirty years, I cannot deny that he had a great wealth of knowledge. I never came across a Sanskrit scholar who dared to talk in front of him in Sanskrit. Having studied the *Yoga Sutra* seven times with him, I realized that he could play with the Sanskrit words in the way a good flutist can play the flute. And what is more, he was an extempore poet. He had such a foundation in *Vedic* chanting that when priests came to our house they would chant in an entirely different way in his presence than they normally did. When we performed the sacred thread ceremony for my two sons, the ceremony that normally takes about fifteen minutes took three days. He was very particular that the prescribed rituals be followed in totality.

Very often, during the years I studied with him, I had the occasion to question him on different schools of Indian thought such as *Buddhism*, *Nyaya*, *Mimamsa*, *Jainism*, and so on. He knew the relevant texts by heart. If, for instance, you asked him to speak about *Buddhism*, you would be left with the impression that he was a *Buddhist* himself. I think I can safely say that there were few of his contemporaries who were as well-educated in the ancient disciplines as him.

There was one striking aspect of his teaching. Whenever I asked him where he had got a certain piece of information, he would always say, "I learnt this from my teacher." Later I realized that a lot of what he had to say was based on his experiences, but he would never acknowledge that. He would say, "I don't say anything. I close my eyes and it is the *guru* in me who says those things."

Another feature of his teaching was his keen sense of observation. Often, he would be seated on a chair reading a newspaper and simultaneously teaching *asana*. It would seem as if he was not paying any attention to the student, but the observations he would make about that student's practice were amazing. As my mother would say, he never saw with his eyes. He always saw with his eyes closed.

I never had much connection with Krishnamacharya, as a father. It was as my teacher that I always related to him. I was much closer to my mother. He did all that he had to do for me as a father—he helped me in my education, he would write to me when he was travelling, he gave me money to buy a cycle or a watch . . . and yet, my connection to him as a teacher was stronger.

Anybody in his position would have definitely made a lot of money. He was, after all, a teacher to no less a person than the *Maharaja* of Mysore. What I admire most about him, is that he never took advantage of his position. When the *Yoga Shala* at Mysore had to be closed after the Independence, he had practically no money. If he had wanted to, he could have very easily secured his future when he had been a teacher at the palace. This is one of the greatest lessons I learnt from my father—to never be a slave of your student.

What remains very strong in my memory was that when I observed him teaching, he would never impose his personal beliefs on his students. Whether *Muslim, Christian,* or *Parsi,* his communication with them always related to their respective belief systems. Always respect the person in front of you. This was another valuable teaching I received from my father. To each person who came to him, he spoke in terms of what he or she related to. With Balasaraswathi, the famous dancer, the focus was *bhakti* (devotion), with Semmangudi Srinivasa Iyer, the icon of the music world, it was music that he discussed. He never insisted that his students necessarily worship God or adapt their beliefs to his. This was a remarkable trait and one that each of us must strive to emulate. 🙶 🙶

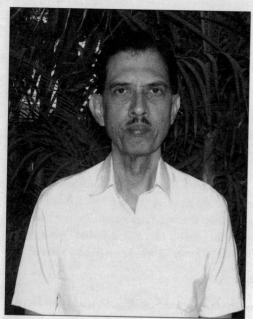

U Suresh Rao in his garden.

U Suresh Rao

Suresh Rao came in contact with his teacher Krishnamacharya in the 1960s and has been a regular practitioner of yoga since then. He is a top chartered accountant by profession and has been an audit consultant for many corporations in India. Suresh Rao is one of the trustees of the Krishnamacharya Yoga Mandiram.

My first meeting with *Sri* Krishnamacharya was through a close friend of mine who learnt yoga under him, and in whose sister's house he was a tenant. I was in my thirties and wished to improve my general health condition.

At first glance, Krishnamacharya's personality was rather awesome—an imposing figure, especially with his caste mark prominently drawn on his forehead, stern, and with a sparkling face. There were no exchange of pleasantries, no courtesies. He came straight to the point and asked me, "What is your problem? What do you want?" At that point I practically had to think up something to say, more to get him interested in me. He asked me to lie down and said he'd examine me. He took my pulse at several points—at my wrists, just below my chest, just above my ankle, on either side of my neck and on the sides of my forehead. Hindsight tells me that he did not require the patient to tell him his/her problem. He could make an assessment based on his own examination. He did not tell me his observations. He merely asked me to come back on a certain date the next month. This whole interaction intrigued me.

On ascertaining my desire to learn, he began to teach me. The yoga classes would start and end with a prayer to the Almighty and to the *Guru*. Noticing me religiously taking down notes on the procedure of doing *asanas*, he asked me, "Are you going to write a book?" It was almost a suggestion. But at that point, the notes were more so that I did not miss out on any important instruction. I was also given a powder (prepared by Krishnamacharya) to be taken along with milk, honey, and ghee every morning for a month, to clear my chest. No money was charged for this powder.

Gradually, after a month or two, the equation between us started to change and he became friendlier. From being extremely matter of fact and formal, he became pleasant and friendly. He always greeted you with a captivating smile. He would demonstrate the *asana* before asking me to do it, in spite of being close to eighty at that time. He was always very careful in prescribing *asanas*. For instance, the first time I did *Sirsasana*, he asked me to do it against the wall, though I was confident of doing it without any support. If I felt any discomfort in doing any *asana*, it would promptly be stopped or altered.

An extraordinary thing about how he supervised the class was that he would know the number of 'rounds' of breathing I had done in my *asanas*, even though he would be either not present physically in the room, or would be reading a book. The monthly fees for the classes were to be placed near the *padukas* of his *guru*.

He expected discipline of a high order both in regularity and punctuality. Classes would be held at odd times, sometimes at 6:30 a.m. and sometimes at 5:00 p.m. When I postponed a class by a day as I was flying to Hyderabad and returning the same day, he advised me to avoid taking two air flights on the same day.

When I took a short break with his permission, because of a stye in my eye, he chided me for stopping all *asana* practices. He said, I ought to have stopped practicing only *Sirsasana*.

193

Any student who was not serious was packed off, never mind that he was a VIP. If a student came to the morning class after a late night, he would promptly notice it in the way the exercises were done, and he would immediately stop the class for that day.

He was a stickler for punctuality. On an occasion when I came a few minutes late for an evening class he said, "You are late. No class today." I learnt from this incident never to be late not only for future yoga classes, but also with respect to my professional engagements.

After a few years, he surprised me by saying that I need not come for any more classes. I was surprised by the suddenness and timing of his instruction. He said this at a point in my life when the fees paid were a considerable percentage of my net income and the discontinuance helped me. I had never discussed the state of my finances with anybody, but *Sri* Krishnamacharya somehow was aware of this.

Certain extraordinary cases—my mother, a widow, was past sixty and frailly built. She often had bouts of giddiness, which none of the Allopathic doctors in Chennai, Mumbai, Bangalore, or Manipal could cure. Within two months of yoga practice under *Sri* Krishnamacharya, she became all right. He chided her when she tried to take umbrage under old age to avoid doing some *asanas* saying, "You are the age of my daughter. How can you give such an excuse when I am watering the garden with a water-can at my age?"

My nephew, who used to get acute stomachache on the morning of an exam (which problem Allopathy could not cure), was cured of his ailment by *Sri* Krishnamacharya. In fact, when it came to young children he was extremely indulgent and not the strict disciplinarian that I spoke of earlier.

Krishnamacharya had one unique trait. He never said "no" to any student, no matter how serious the problem was. He would never say, "Let me see if I can help" or "I will try." He was confidence personified when dealing with patients.

I was invited as a trustee of KYM, to attend the *homam* organised at KYM's first premises on St. Mary's Road, to mark the formal inauguration of the KYM. When I reached KYM, it was around ten in the morning as I had to finish some work at my office first.

Desikachar said, "You must act as the *Yajamanam* [chief functionary of the ritual]." I refused, since I was not appropriately dressed and felt that Desikachar, as the Managing Trustee, would be the right person. My excuse of being inappropriately dressed was overruled. This surprised me. Inspite of being such an orthodox person, Krishnamacharya had invited me to be a part of the ceremonies, even though I was inappropriately dressed. Another thing that surprised me was that *Vedic* hymns like *Rudram* and *Camakam* were being chanted in what I had thought would be a purely *Vaisnavite* affair, given Krishnamacharya's background. Such instances only go to emphasize Krishnamacharya's magnanimity and acceptance of traditions other than his own.

A well-known Sanskrit scholar, Krishnamurthy Sastrigal, who was suffering from a problem with his shoulder, wanted to meet Krishnamacharya. This was about a month before Krishnamacharya's hundredth birthday. When Krishnamurthy Sastrigal came into the room, Krishnamacharya offered him a seat—the traditional flat wooden plank (*manai*). However, Krishnamurthy Sastrigal was a little hesistant to sit before Krishnamacharya. Krishnamacharya then convinced Sastrigal that as he was a guest, he was entitled to this honor. This entire conversation was in Sanskrit. Krishnamacharya then gave Sastrigal some *Tailam* (special herbal oil), after reciting certain Sanskrit verses while holding the *Tailam*. Krishnamurthy Sastrigal was so touched by Krishnamacharya's kind gestures, that when asked to officiate at Krishnamacharya's centenary celebrations, he readily agreed. Krishnamurthy Sastrigal thought that it was an honor conferred on him. One hundred and eight eminent priests were present—indeed a Herculean effort. Sastrigal attributed the attendance of such eminent priests of the highest calibre to Krishnamacharya's magnetic personality and not to his own organising capabilities.

As Krishnamacharya's birthday drew near, I thought hard about what one could give a hundred-year-old man, who had no worldly desires. A few weeks before his birthday, I came across a beautiful picture of Lord *Rama* (of Vadavur Temple) which I enlarged and delivered at his house. When I was later called along with a few others like AMM Arunachalam, the first thing he said was, "Suresh Rao has brought *Rama* to me." I was touched by his warmth and yet a little embarrassed that he chose to honor me on that occasion even before the other eminent seniors who were present.

There are many such moments that stay in my memory, and I could easily write on and on. But, one thing is sure. Krishnamacharya was a teacher par excellence, and it is unfortunate that the wealth of knowledge that he had acquired has still to be fully exploited by the world.

With his *Yoga Siddhi* (yogic powers) and through his teachings, he was able to help so many people, including foreigners, physically, mentally, and spiritually. He lived a very disciplined life and was so affectionate to his *sisyas* (students). He was so full of *Satguna* (good qualities). I have never met such an authority on Yoga, *Veda*, *Ayurveda*, *Mimamsa*, and *Vedanta* as Krishnamacharya. He was indeed a great being. 🙶

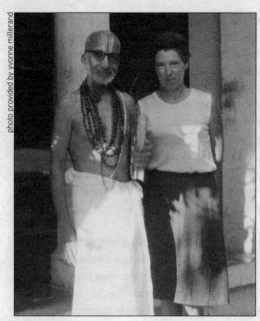

Yvonne Millerand with Krishnamacharya.

Yvonne Millerand

Yvonne Millerand was a sportswoman in the early part of her life, and she met Krishnamacharya in the 1960s. She went on to teach yoga and was instrumental in creating the French School of Yoga. She also authored a book titled *Practical Guide of Hatha Yoga.* She continued her studies with Desikachar after Krishnamacharya's death and had returned to India many times before she passed away in 2007.

I started practicing yoga in 1952, under the guidance of Lucien Ferrer. There were few students at first, but very quickly their numbers increased. Lucien Ferrer had a gift for healing and was being assailed by requests, which made teaching yoga more and more difficult for him. Being one of his oldest pupils, he asked me to take charge of lessons for him. And so, I became his assistant without really being prepared for it.

Teaching sort of grew on me, so I reread my anatomy books to check the exact roles of muscles and viscera to be sure of avoiding any mistakes. This lasted for twelve years. When Lucien Ferrer died in 1964, I found myself with no more instructions for teaching other than what I had learnt from him. I had been giving private lessons to Mrs. Jean Klein, who became a good friend. She had visited India several times and we would often talk about her experiences. Her daughters Nita and Christine and Christine's husband Jean-Georges Henrotte were all very fond of India.

Christine was studying *Bharathanatyam*, the classical dance form of South India. Jean-Georges Henrotte was a doctor who had stayed with his wife for two years in India, for professional reasons. They had met *Sri* Krishnamacharya in Madras, and Dr. Henrotte was enthusiastic about the quality of his teaching.

When Mrs. Klein told her family that I was looking for a master in yoga, Jean-Georges Henrotte said that as far as he was concerned, he knew only one person who actually deserved that status. He urged me to go to Madras, because the master was nearly seventy-six years old, and might not be accepting students for very long. I wrote to *Sri* Krishnamacharya, and many letters were exchanged between us before I actually went to India.

Some conditions were stipulated about my stay. I was to promise not to eat eggs, meat, or fish. Of course, I accepted. I was also happy that Christine would be in India at the same time. I finally received a very warm and welcoming letter from Madras, and left at the end of August. Christine had preceded me, reserving my hotel room, and best of all, getting me an appointment with the Master for the 3rd of September, 1964 at 5:00 p.m. She came with me and presented me to the Master at that first meeting.

He was sitting on a flight of steps. He greeted us and then had us enter the classroom. After a moment of silence, sitting on an armchair, he said, "Show me what you can do."

I was very impressed but managed to execute everything that came to my mind—front flexing, backward extension, doing the splits on both sides, rotations, *Pascimatanasana*, *Ardha Padmasana*, *Sarvangasana*, *Sirsasana*, and many others. I sat down and looked at him. Suddenly, he asked me, "Why have you left your master?" Christine and I answered at the same time,"He is dead, sir."

In English, difficult for me to understand, he said, "You know nothing. You don't know how to breathe and you hop about like a sparrow! Come back on Friday at 5:00 p.m., not before and not later."

I was there, just on time. Giving me several lessons per week, he started with simple *asana* practice. I was to ally breathing and movement. Breathing was to rule the movement of the arms, the slower the breathing, the slower the movement. Every *asana* was to be repeated at least four times.

At the end of one hour of class in the sitting position, I had learned to make the sound of *Ujjayi* and be able to distinguish it from the nasal sound. That allowed me to start the simplest *pranayama—Ujjayi Anuloma* and *Ujjayi Viloma.*

Krishnamacharya often told me to "high up the chest," so that by raising my ribcage, I could inspire the flow of air to the base of my lungs. After that, he insisted on expiration, using the abdominal and perineal muscles. To inhale and exhale is natural, but by inserting pauses, everything is changed. The control that is exercised feels like the assertion of life and gives the impression of living better, by managing the breathing and blood circulation, which are linked. This is what I felt.

After some *asanas*, he taught me the role of counter-*asana*, the role of which is to remove certain negative consequences. He taught me many *asanas* I never knew. He never imposed their Sanskrit names on me and whenever possible, he would use the English language—"bed pose, hill pose, shoulderstanding, head-standing . . . and so on." On the other hand, he taught me all the Sanskrit names of *pranayama.*

After some time, he would take my pulse before and after a lesson. My pulse rate was not to go over 65 pulsations per minute, so that he would be sure that my breathing had harmoniously followed the effort during *asana* practice.

Time went by very quickly. Towards the end of my stay, Krishnamacharya insisted especially on two *asanas* and their variations—*Sarvangasana* and *Sirsasana*. He would ask me to stay in these postures, first for fifteen minutes and then gradually, for twenty minutes. He wanted me to equalize the number of breaths in each case. I have never really been able to do this for *Sarvangasana*, feeling more at ease with *Sirsasana*. What I preferred were two types of *pranayama—Nadi Sodhana* and *Pratiloma*. I cannot describe all that I learnt from him, but I have never forgotten all that.

I still have my last experience before I left Madras, printed on my memory. After a few *asanas*, Krishnamacharya asked me to do the headstand and stay there for thirty minutes and to count my breaths. He stayed in the classroom, watching the clock until the time was over. I was very busy trying to keep my balance and to count the number of breaths. I put my fingers one after another on my occiput at every inspiration so that when I had used my ten fingers, I knew I had completed ten breaths.

As I finished my thirty-sixth exhalation, Krishnamacharya told me to lie down on the floor for a while. I felt good, but as I went out of the classroom, into the daylight, an extraordinary thing happened. I was surrounded by a blue light, as if I was in the sky. Around me I could not see anything else but blue. I still wonder how I found my way back to the hotel, probably like a well-programmed robot. I sat down in my room, my mind empty, not thinking, not moving. Slowly, the blueness faded and disappeared. A question rose to my mind, "What happened to me?" I had practically done one breath per minute. Was it the *asana*, or the slowness of my breath that had produced this vacuity in my mind? My mistake has been that I did not dare to tell Krishnamacharya about this experience during my next lesson.

On my last day in India, I brought a basket of fruits and a flower garland for my Master. He gave me a diploma and granted me permission to transmit his lessons to others. His wife and son were present which was a great honor for me. My stay in India was the greatest adventure of my life.

My relationship with Krishnamacharya changed a lot during the course of my stay. I did what I was asked to without asking any questions. If I did not understand the Sanskrit name of any *asana*, the master would say it and I would repeat after him. He was hard to please, but always fair. Gradually, I understood better the words he used. He would speak softly, and I began to feel more at ease with him. A sort of intimacy grew between us, and he seemed happy when he saw me. I eventually dared to ask him,"How does a *yogi* react when facing poverty on the streets?" I had seen a dead man lying on a street, totally ignored by those who passed by. He answered, "I take care of those who are near me. Where I can do something efficient, such as feed or heal the ones sleeping at my door, I will do it. For others, I pray."

We used to talk during the short breaks after the end of *asana* practice and before beginning *pranayama*. Once I dared to ask him what he thought about the *cakras*, for everybody was talking about them in Europe at that time. He said, "You must not touch the three lower *cakras*, for they are dependent on one another. At the front of the head, *Ajna* symbolizes the conscience, on top of the head, *Sahasrara* is symbolic of perfect knowledge, but the most important one is at the heart." He did not mention the throat *cakra*, which surprised me. The lessons went on.

I was really moved one day, when I was doing a lengthy *pranayama* practice with Krishnamacharya sitting in front of me in a rattan chair, his eyes closed. I felt then an urge to open my eyes and look at him. An image forced itself on me—a black rigid figure, around which a golden light was shining, an aura full of sweet love, which hit me directly and wrapped me all over, as if the master had lifted me to a new state of consciousness. I was very moved and enchanted. Nevertheless, I finished my practice. No word was said, but I never forgot that experience

Krishnamacharya trusted me enough to suggest that I should use the name of *"Narayana"* during *pranayama*. He pronounced it, stressing on the letter "r," making me repeat it until he was satisfied with my pronunciation. He then said, "This sacred name belongs to my tradition. You have to find in your own culture the name which you want to invoke in the depth of your heart." I was free from all influence and thanked him for this.

On my return, I found a classroom and my faithful students. Everybody was so eager to hear about India and the Master. What I taught was literally a revolution for the students. The *asanas* were either dynamic

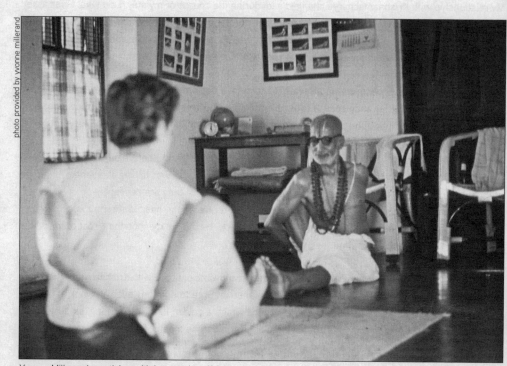

photo provided by yvonne millerand

Yvonne Millerand practicing with her teacher, Krishnamacharya.

or static which they had never done before. The nasal sound and "*Ujjayi* breathing" were unknown to them. It took them several months to adapt to such a string of novelties.

I wished that working this way, the students would become more interiorised and that the fusion of mind and body would bring them to a better understanding, being less materialistic, aiming to institute inner calm, and helping them to discover what was most important in their lives. The work I did under the care of Krishnamacharya magnified my physical and psychic sensitivity.

As soon as the students were lying on the carpet, I could feel their inner states. I knew at once when they were sad, worried, sick, or disturbed. It allowed me to speak to them and organize my lessons accordingly for the whole class. Each lesson was different. I respected the "*Vinyasa*" technique of preparation for an *asana* and then leading to its execution. The various problems faced by my students led me to find measures to help them overcome their difficulties.

Krishnamacharya changed my life by admitting me as a student. I think of him as a living entity who continues to inspire me. His wisdom and patience are still alive in my mind. Just as a child can love his/her school master, I loved him with all the respect due to him. 〞

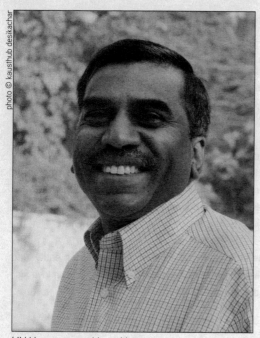

photo © kausthub desikachar

MM Murugappan at his residence.

MM Murugappan

MM Murugappan is Chairman of one of the largest companies in India. He met his teacher, Krishnamacharya, through his uncle, MV Murugappan, and has been a regular practitioner of yoga since the 1980s. He continues his practice with Desikachar and is an advocate of yoga in the business community. He is actively involved in many social projects in and around Chennai.

My first impression of T. Krishnamacharya, and one that stays with me till today, is of being totally awestruck by this elderly man, seated on a verandah, who addressed me in a deep voice. It was around 1981–82, and I used to suffer from chronic eosinophilia. Working in a factory did nothing to improve my condition. I had tried a whole range of treatments, and finally, my uncle, MV Murugappan took me to meet Krishnamacharya. He asked my uncle about me, and then told me to return after a week. Being in a line of work that dealt with scientifically proven theories and medical practices, I always set great store by fact-based information. It was in such a frame of mind that I returned to see Krishnamacharya after a week. He again asked me to come back after another week. I was a little frustrated, but at the same time I was so awestruck by this man, that I never felt the urge to question him. It was only after the third week that he took me on as a student.

Then, I was perhaps too young and inexperienced to comprehend the significance of making me return week after week. But now, I find myself emulating Krishnamacharya's example. If anybody wants my time for some purpose, I tend to first test their genuineness and the degree of interest they display. Today, I realize that only if you are totally committed to and interested in something will you give it your fullest, and this is what Krishnamacharya wanted to see in me.

Under his guidance, I felt my health improve progressively. I used to play competitive squash in those days. Somehow, I never picked up the courage to tell him about this, but he found out in his own way. He never stopped me from playing, perhaps because he knew how much I enjoyed it. Rather, he modified my exercise to take care of that requirement. Once, I had not practiced for about three weeks. The first thing he asked me when he saw me was, "Has it been three weeks since you practiced?" I was dumbfounded at his perception.

Another incident comes to mind. My exercise time with Krishnamacharya was once a week in the evening. Often, he'd sit with his eyes closed while I did my practice. It would appear as if he was deep in sleep, but if I stopped my practice to see if he had anything to say he would immediately ask me to proceed.

His room was next to the terrace, with a bathroom attached. On one occasion, when I was practicing, I heard the sound of water overflowing from a bucket. I got up from my practice to turn the tap off and carry the bucket, but he stopped me and said, "You continue your practice. Do you think I cannot carry that myself?" Then he proceeded to carry that bucket full of water himself. At that time he must have been at least ninety-four years old. By that time, I must say that I was totally taken up with (and in complete awe of) this man.

Whenever we began a practice session, it would always be with a prayer to *Narayana*, a prayer that forms a part of my life to this day. It was only after two years that I even picked up the courage to have a conversation with him. He was quite surprised that I could write in Hindi and Sanskrit in spite of being a Tamilian and he modified my practice timings so that I could learn some *slokas* from him. What was amazing was that for any query of mine on absolutely any subject, he would give his point of view and recite a relevant *sloka* from various texts like the *Bhagavad Gita*, *Mahabharatha*, and *Gita Govinda*, complete with its contextual significance and meaning. It was from him that I learnt how to look deep within any situation or concept, and to relate to that situation or concept.

He was extremely discrete and would never discuss a person's state of health or attitude with anybody else. This touched me greatly, because I was after all another student and he need not have shown me such a degree of respect. Looking back, I realize that this quality of mutual respect between two individuals is something I learnt from him. In dealing with sensitive issues he was very measured and accurate in what he said. In some cases he would remain silent and I grew to realize that those moments of silence held greater meaning than when he answered my queries. So much so that, even today when I meet and converse with people, I tend to look for what is unsaid. It never occurred to me to ask him the reason for his silence, but I realize that my query was either irrelevant or did not deserve a reply. And another thing that struck me about him, was that he never told me what I wanted to hear. Often, I meet people who will say many things just to please one. Not him. He would never insist that I had to do something or concur with his point of view. He would only say, "this is how I feel" or "this is my experience."

After the second year or so, we became really good friends, and remained so until he passed away. In fact, when he was in hospital towards his last days, I could never bring myself to go and see him there. I lost my father very early in life. It really helped to have a person like Krishnamacharya to speak to. In my early professional years, I benefited greatly from this friendship with a man like him who had my well-being at heart, and yet who was exterior to my immediate family circle. I don't quite remember just when we crossed that threshold and became more than just a teacher and student. It took a lot of courage, at least for me and although I never got over my awe of him, I am glad we were friends.

While I always treasured my association with Krishnamacharya, it was only much later after he was no more that I learnt that my friendship had also meant a lot to him. What began with me seeking help for a medical problem, grew into a great affinity. I believed in him unconditionally and valued greatly his friendship, but it never occurred to me to ask him what he felt because of the sheer awe with which I regarded him. Later, when Desikachar asked me to be on the Board of Trustees, he told me that his father had specifically asked him to involve me in the activities of the Mandiram. He told me that he had never seen Krishnamacharya looking forward so eagerly to a student coming to see him, as he had done with me. And yet, in spite of that degree of closeness, there was never the slightest compromise on courtesy or reverence towards him.

Today, it is unfortunate that there is no one of his stature with whom to have a conversation. I think I was just very fortunate to have even known him, and I am glad that my association with his family continues to this day. I have the utmost respect for Desikachar and value what I have learnt from him, but I realize that what draws me towards yoga, towards heritage and using the strength of our culture, was my interaction with Krishnamacharya.

Throughout the time I knew him, between 1982 and 1989, he would be the person I would always go to see, whenever anything good happened in my family like the birth of a child. I am a person who never goes to a temple by program. For me it was enough if I could just speak to Krishnamacharya and get his blessings. He was by far one of the greatest influences in my life and now when I introspect, I realize that what made me hold him in such awe was that palpable relationship between knowledge and wisdom that I saw in him.

Those days, I would never miss a single class with him, unless it was absolutely impossible to attend. There were times when I would go for my practice with him even if I felt unwell. On such occasions he would offer me a special preparation made of almond, ghee, and sugar. One day, he asked me to bring my wife along and taught her how to make it. This was an act that touched me greatly.

He could be short-tempered and he would make no compromise when it came to doing things properly. Yet he was always open to adaptability. Even today, when I have held a rigid stand on some professional issue, I wonder if I might have perhaps achieved better results had I been a little more flexible. This was one thing I learnt from him, which I realize the significance of more today than I did then.

His depth of knowledge never ceased to amaze me. He was orthodox in his ways, and yet aware of sociological issues. He would never compromise on his principles but he was liberal enough to accept that societal changes were inevitable and would insist that if one stuck to his or her principles, it was possible to influence these changes. I realize the import of what he said only now after so many years of introspection. When Desikachar and I sometimes discuss our experiences with Krishnamacharya, I realize that what he said about practically any issue, continues to be relevant today.

He taught me that one never needed to compromise on one's principles. From him I imbibed the ability to discern good from bad and right from wrong. He taught me to set high personal standards. When you continuously strive for improvement, you tend to associate with similar people. And hence, the few people whom I can today count as my best friends are in the normal course very difficult to deal with. The more I reflect, the more it reinforces what I learnt from him. He is one of the most important teachers I have had in life. Today, after so much reflection and introspection I continue to feel the relevance of what he taught me. Even today, when I meet any others who have been associated with Krishnamacharya, our conversation will automatically drift to a discussion about some aspect or attribute of Krishnamacharya. That was the power of his teaching and the influence he exerted on those who were fortunate enough to be associated with him.

I only wish I could have known him longer. I have his photo in my study and never a day goes by that does not begin with the prayer to Lord *Narayana* that he taught me. Every time I go to visit Desikachar, to discuss any matter, I automatically go to the *Sannidhi* first. I have all his writings, which I often read and reread, not so much in search of knowledge as to reinforce my belief that Krishnamacharya is still present with me. He was like a magnet, attracting you, not out of any compulsion but out of reverence and respect for an outstandingly evolved individual, the likes of whom you rarely meet in a lifetime. " "

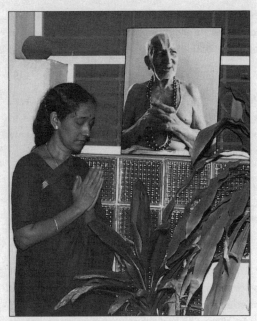

Mala Srivatsan chanting at her home.

Mala Srivatsan

Mala Srivatsan met her teacher, Krishnamacharya, in the early 1980s and has been a student of yoga since then. She was one of the first female students to be taught chanting by Krishnamacharya. She has been a teacher at Krishnamacharya Yoga Mandiram since 1990 and served as its Executive Trustee from 1991 to 2001. She continues her practice with Desikachar and lives in Chennai with her husband and two children.

Experiences with *Mahatmas* (great people) are stunning and it is very difficult to put into words my experience with my *acarya*, T Krishnamacharya. The experience stays and words become a weak attempt of expression. To be very truthful, even the person who has experienced such an interaction only starts to appreciate it as he/she moves on because at that point of time one is unable to absorb the feeling in full.

His simplicity, humility, spontaneity, wisdom, and over and above everything else, his compassion were directly and unmistakably experienced in his presence. In plain English the only thing I can say is that I loved him a lot, but I really wonder if even this is an adequate expression of my feelings. The closest that I can think of is the Sanskrit term, "*Prema,*" which literally means devotion, that is rooted in love. Even now, when I think of him I can only think of that love. To rationalize it in any other way is superfluous.

When I was Krishnamacharya's student, I didn't know anything about him. It was only when I undertook to write his biography* that I learned of his virtuosity. Perhaps, if I had known then of all his accomplishments, I would have been scared of him. This ignorance was, in a way, bliss, as it did not interfere with the absolute joy that I experienced in his presence.

He played many different roles at every stage in my life. He was more like a mother, compassionate, understanding, and always giving before one asked for it. Aren't these the qualities of a mother? When it came to discipline he was like a father. In a lighter mood, he would debate with me on some subject. I would suddenly feel that we were talking like friends, but most of the time he was undoubtedly my *acarya* guiding me for the future.

When I first met him in 1980, he was close to ninety and I was just twenty-three. But he never had any problem relating to me, as he came down to my level of communication. His passion to communicate perfectly and to see the desired effect on the student was his only aim. He was like a mirror and would reflect with the same intensity of approach that was shown to him. His teaching was a demonstration of purity, tolerance, grace, compassion, and intense spiritual relationship. It was not that he was easy-going either. I realized that he got what he wanted out of you.

Only an *acarya* can influence and conduct your life along a suitable path. What was significant was that he embraced my whole family and drew my husband and children also towards him. His love and blessings are always with my family. It was because of that family involvement that I was able to serve at KYM in the later years. My husband, who was a fanatical Western exercise addict, switched to yoga under his guidance, and even today he tells our children that yoga made him a better person in many ways. In fact, it was Krishnamacharya who named my children. I am sure that whatever their beliefs and attitudes are now, they will grow up to be what he wished them to be. There are not many *acaryas* like him who will care for an individual's entire family. By entire family, I even include my brothers, sisters, niece, and nephews. They have all been under his healing touch.

---

* Mala Srivatsan wrote the first biography of T Krishnamacharya. It was published by the Krishnamacharya Yoga Mandiram in 1997. It has been out of print since 2001 and is one of the main inspirations for this book.

There is no strength like love to keep you moving, and it was this love that I experienced from him. The feeling of wanting to take care of you was so intensely felt in his presence. Many people speak about his accomplishments, and his great sense of discipline, but somehow I feel that he was more than all that. He was more than just a human being. Often, we need somebody to emulate and the presence of such a person can make all the difference in one's life. To me, he was and is everything. What I learnt during my growing up with him was to just do my duty without expecting anything in return (I am still making an attempt at this). He taught me never to take any decision in anger or haste. He believed in leaving everything to Lord *Narayana*.

Coming from a traditional religious background, I was well-acquainted with the Hindu concept of God, but through him, that kind of total and selfless devotion was reinforced in my life. Nothing was more important to him than devotion and dedication to God. This devotion was uppermost in all that he taught. When he taught me *pranayama* he said, "When you inhale, remember that this breath was given to you by God, and when you exhale, remember that it goes back to him." He never set any conditions, but what he said then has always stayed with me. All that he taught was never a mere reiteration of an ancient text. His teaching was suffused with *bhakti*. He learnt from his teachers in a certain way. He lived that way, and he taught the same way.

The question of how and why I first met Krishnamacharya, seems unimportant in the face of the depth of my feelings for him.

For the record, I was a severe asthmatic and was on medicines to control my wheezing. I was newly married then, my sister told me about him, and I went to meet him. He asked me if he could examine me and took my pulse at three different points. He asked me if I would agree to stop my allopathic medications and asked me to follow a certain diet. He said that he would begin my practice after a week. His ethics made him wonder if I was ready to follow his treatment or if I needed to consult my husband. I did not hesitate. Just to be in his presence filled me with confidence. This unshakeable faith made me agree immediately. And at that age, he himself prepared for me a certain *Ayurvedic* medicine. He began teaching me after a week. On the second day, I stopped wheezing. I can't explain this scientifically, but I know that it was his confidence that he could help me, and mine in him, that cured me.

After a few months, he told me that he wanted me to become a yoga teacher. At this time I did not know even a single word from any text on yoga. He said, "I want you to teach." So the preparation started by teaching me the *Hatha Yoga Pradipika*. He taught selective sections of this text. Then he moved on to teach the *Yoga Sutra*. I studied only two chapters from him. He taught me the *Yoga Sutra* based on his own commentary the *Yogavalli*, and until I joined the KYM as a diploma student, I thought that this was the only way this text could be learnt and understood.

One day, he said, "Tell the people near your house that you teach yoga." I did so, and two people came to me asking for lessons. I did not know a thing about teaching yoga or even how to examine somebody. He told me to brief him about their problems. I spoke to them, and then went back to him. He would question me about their body structures, eating habits, etc. Sitting there, he drew up a course for them, which I taught as per his instructions. Based on my observations, he would then alter their courses. That is how I first began to teach yoga.

Later, I joined the KYM to do my diploma, so that I could teach with more confidence. The institute gave me an opportunity to learn and serve and this could not have come without his wish and blessings. One can never repay an *acarya* for what you have received. Whatever you do is but a minuscule recognition of the wealth of compassion that you have received.

After five years, he said that he wanted me to learn chanting. We began with a passage from the *Mahanaryana Upanisad*. Later, I learnt that I was the first woman to learn chanting from him. Even those chants were never taught to me for the sake of learning. He would always select chants that prayed for well-being and that promoted mental and physical health. He would pick passages and excerpts from various texts that he thought I personally needed. My last lessons with him were from the *Bhagavad Gita,* thirteenth chapter, which speaks about the highest knowledge and Self-realization. His lifetime did not permit him to fulfill what he wanted for me, but there is absolutely no doubt in my mind the he will complete it.

To look back, he has guided me through my life, not just in a theoretical sense. Beginning with a focus on health and fitness, he taught me the *Hatha Yoga Pradipika*. Then he moved to the *Yoga Sutra*, which deals with the mind. My chanting lessons were calculated to enhance my physical, mental, and spiritual well-being. And in teaching me the *Bhagavad Gita*, he taught me that it was important to go beyond the physical body and to keep progressing till you realize the greater self within you. At that time, I had neither the maturity nor the experience to reflect upon and draw from his teachings or to even question him. People ask me today, why I never asked him any questions. The fact is, it never occurred to me to ask him questions. I only knew to relate to that all-encompassing love that engulfed me in his presence. Perhaps it was quite stupid of me, but I was quite content and even today, I have no regrets.

He guided me then, and he continues to guide me now. There can be only a few such *acaryas* who would want to protect you under the umbrella of their compassion, expecting nothing in return but your progress. You have nothing to give back, but at the very least, we can receive graciously.

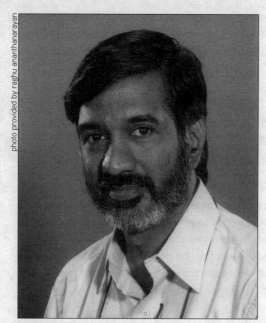
photo provided by raghu ananthanarayan

Raghu Ananthanarayanan in his workplace.

Raghu Ananthanarayan

Raghu Ananthanarayanan met Krishnamacharya through his own teacher, Desikachar, in the 1970s. Raghu was an undergraduate student when he became interested in yoga and has been one of its strongest advocates since then. He was a teacher at the Krishnamacharya Yoga Mandiram, before becoming a management consultant offering business solutions inspired by Indian wisdom and tradition. He lives in Chennai with his wife, who is an architect.

Preamble

I have sat down to write this paper and found it very difficult to do justice to the task of honoring my *Guru*. I have decided to chronicle my transformation through my association with Desikachar and his father. However, a few disclaimers may be appropriate. The work that I do in facilitating group encounters involves a fair amount of "self disclosure" in the participants. The dialogue proceeds through a slow but meaningful exchange of one's inner reality. I feel that I will be able to remain authentic to myself, respect my *Guru* and the reader simultaneously by using a similar method. I seek the reader's patience and to bear with me and read what follows as a "story in the first person" and not as an attempt to glorify myself.

My first meeting

Desikachar often refers to my first meeting with him. Prabhakar (my friend) had taken me across to meet him since I was keen on learning Yoga. Desikachar describes me as "tense, intense, and desperate." Those were some of the most difficult days of my life. I was deeply hurt inwardly by what I experienced as my father's betrayal of me. In my workspace, I had to rebuild my life after the family business had gone into a sudden and dramatic collapse. I was in the early years of my marriage. We had an infant son and a second child was on the way. The business collapse meant that I was left with a legacy of an unsaleable small scale business and a complex tangle of legal and financial crises from the larger business. The banks were threatening to turn the matter into a "criminal investigation." Without a rebuilding of my inner psyche and self, there was no way I was going to find the ability to confront the problems ramming down my door!

The first spark of hope was kindled in me through a meeting I had with J Krishnamurti. In that meeting, I recounted to him my turmoil, my anger, my need to seek retribution, and my feelings of betrayal. After listening to me for nearly an hour, J Krishnamurti just said, "Sir, your anger and inner violence is not the issue. You are very hurt and raw from the feeling of being let down by your father. Deal with that."

I met Desikachar soon after this. In a sense, a door had been opened, but I had not dared to take the first steps on the road to an inner healing. I spent almost ten years studying and teaching yoga. The contact with Desikachar and his father has transformed deeply.

My first yoga lesson

After initially putting me off, Desikachar accepted me as his student. I will never forget the first yoga class I had with him. I clearly recall those days when my mind was literally clouded. I would experience myself as seated in a crouched posture in a dark room. Very simply and directly, Desikachar put me through the *asana* course. Then he sat me down to do a simple *pranayama*. Slowly, a small bright spot of light appeared within me, and by the time I completed the 16 or 20 breaths of simple inhale and exhale, this light had spread through me. Slowly and softly, I was helped to take my first step. Obviously, I was completely hooked.

I am introduced to the *Yogacarya*

When I started learning with Desikachar, it was in a room upstairs that does not exist now in his home. On the way up or down, one would encounter his father seated in the verandah. There was an unmistakable presence though the *Yogacarya* was only reading a paper in the morning!

Yoacarya Krishnamacharya was a familiar person in my maternal family. My aunt, who is afflicted with polio, had learnt yoga from him in the '50s when the *Yogacarya* had just come to Chennai. I have heard from her the stories of how he would come home and teach my aunt with great kindness. She always mentioned that while others felt he was very stern, with her, the *Yogacarya* was very gentle and compassionate. Some of my cousins were long-time disciples of the *Yogacarya*, but I had only heard of him and never met him.

The first time I saw the *Yogacarya*, his presence confirmed in my mind the awe and respect in which he was held at home. It was almost a year after I started lessons with Desikachar that I was formally introduced to the *Yogacarya* in a class. In those days, there was a large thatched room next to the room in which Desikachar took his classes. On Saturday evenings, *Yogacarya* would teach for an hour. The classes always started with about ten minutes of chanting. *Yogacarya* almost always had his eyes closed and sat in a perfect *Padmasana*. Desikachar and sometimes a *shastrigal* (priest) would chant with *Yogacarya*. The effect this had was a calming of the mind and a gradual focusing of one's attention on *Yogacarya*. These classes always had a central theme, the *Bhagavad Gita*, or the *Yoga Sutra* or the meaning of various rituals, or an *Upanisad*. What was very significant to me was the "modernity" or should I say timelessness of the way *Yogacarya* explained the concepts. There were always a few very interesting personal anecdotes that he would share. The time he spent at Manasarovar with Rammohana Brahmachari took shape in one's mind through snippets of experiences he shared from time to time. One story stands out, about learning which stream to drink from (near the caves) at different times since each stream flowed through a part of the forest with different herbs and thus had different effects on the body! Or, the time with the Mysore *Maharaja*, teaching the *Maharaja* horse-riding for example. This hour was profound in its philosophical context, but, simultaneously, it had the evocative quality of listening to a great story unfold.

All this had a very deep impact on me. In the absence of any real dialogue about the meaning of rituals and daily discipline, at home, I had cast off my *punal* (sacred thread) and stopped respecting the tradition. The heady influence of being part of the '60s student rebellion and the "Woodstock" generation made further inroads into my tenuous links with tradition. A small group of us at college did study Aurobindo and Zen Buddhism and debated things amongst ourselves. But this went hand in hand with trying to understand Marx and Marcuse. In the absence of a real teacher to help us, these enquiries were the desperate attempts to make sense of the bewildering world we were entering as young adults. In every one of the Saturday lessons, I found some aspect or the other of my questions and doubts being resolved. By the end of the year, I had starting wearing my "*punal*" again and doing the morning *Sandhyavandanam* (sun ritual). However, I did not at any time find the rational or "modern" part of me at odds with the way *Yogacarya* expounded on the great truths in the *sastras*. Just to illustrate, let me quote an incident from a ew years later. *Yogacarya* would sometimes entertain questions. One of the students raised a question about teaching chanting to women and to non-Hindus. *Yogacarya's* answer still rings in my ears. "Do you accept that He is the *antaryami* of all beings?" he asked. "Do you also accept that the *atma* in each human being is an aspect of the Lord?"

"Of course," said the questioner.

"OM is the word that refers to that infinite intelligence. When that Intelligence already resides within each person, who are you or I to say that the words that revere Him can or cannot be uttered by any one?"

About women the answer was simple. "If the mother is not educated in the scriptures and in Yoga, who will impart it to the children?"

I am invited to teach Yoga

The Yoga Mandiram was just taking birth around the time I was a year or more into learning from Desikachar. Lakshmi and Prabhakar were already teaching. All this was at Desikachar's home and the "upstairs" spaces were getting more and more crowded.

Suddenly, out of the blue, Desikachar asked me one day, "Do you want to teach Yoga?" I said, "Yes," and promptly, a young dancer who needed help with her dance posture was told, "He will teach you!" Here I was a neophyte with a body that was just learning to relax, faced with teaching a dancer with an obviously more flexible body and greater range of movement! After she left, I ventured to ask Desikachar, "How will I be able to teach her?"

"If you think that the form is what you are teaching, you are mistaken. There is a transfer of energy from within. Trust that and trust my choice of you as a teacher," he said.

In the Saturday class, in the midst of his lesson, *Yogacarya* talked about teaching and echoed Desikachar's words. He called the contact between teacher and student a "transfer of power" and said that one must place faith in *Isvara* when one is teaching. I don't think Desikachar asked *Yogacarya* to talk about this, I believe Yogacarya would intuitively respond to the doubts and sincere questions of the students in the class.

Some time later, I was invited to join a small class of Desikachar, Prabhakar, and myself. We met with *Yogacarya* three to four times a week. These classes were an intensive exposition of the *Yoga Sutra* and the *Upanisads*. The mode of this teaching has fascinated me. The class always started with chanting. We had learnt to chant the *Yoga Sutra* with Desikachar. We had also listened to the "overview" of the *Yoga Sutra* in the Saturday classes. So one had a broad idea of the teaching contained in the *Yoga Sutra*. Then *Yogacarya* would take up one *sutra* after the other to explain. Firstly, each word would be explained with its root meanings. Then, an explanation of the whole *sutra*, with parallels drawn from the *Bhagavad Gita* or the *Upanisads*. If a word from the particular sector is repeated in the *Yoga Sutra* later, the differentia tone would be explicated.

The beauty of all this was that the learning one received was always holistic. While I cannot claim to know the "whole" of the text (though I have studied it about four times with *Yogacarya* and Desikachar) and all its ramifications, what was taught was always in well-rounded wholes. Each subsequent exposition therefore expanded the "volume of the sphere." Of course this can keep expanding infinitely, and that's exactly the beauty of this learning. When compared to a "linear" teaching, the "beauty" becomes clear. I studied engineering. But, not only was each aspect taught separately, by an expert, each part was taught in a logical but linear manner. I had to then put all these pieces together and puzzle out the whole picture. I was taught the aspects of engineering, but not taught to be an "engineer" or what it meant to be one!

These classes always had bits of personal anecdotes and each of these also illustrated what it meant to be a yoga teacher. One particular story is about how the *Yogacarya* taught yoga to a *Mulla*. The *Mulla* living in Triplicane requested *Yogacarya*. "It will be embarrassing for me as a leader of my [Muslim] community to come to your place, can you please help me." *Yogacarya* would go to the *Mulla's* house through its back door (in a cycle rickshaw). Soon, the two of them had struck a deep friendship and would discourse on the *Quoran*. We learnt in the course of this story that *Yogacarya* had learnt some of the secrets of breath and *asana* in a book from Afghanistan called *Hakeekattul Insaan*.

Having to teach yoga made one listen more deeply and practice more intensely. Some of the transformations I went through as I healed inwardly are due to this intense engagement with Desikachar and *Yogacarya*. What I found happening to me was that I learnt to let my mind unfold at its will, during the "rest" after a course of yoga. I discovered later that what I was doing was being "a witness." My mind would automatically form images as the mental manifestation of problems that were bothering me. At one point of time, I was very troubled by my relationship with my father and wondering how to resolve it. In one of the "rest" periods, I was struck by the vision of a goat tied to a stake banging its head against a hillock. Slowly, the goat stops the incessant banging of his head, it transforms into a bird, the clasp around the neck falls off, and the bird flies over the hillock! These visions were always accompanied by a deep relaxation of the body as though releasing a grip from the inside.

Though I seldom spoke to Desikachar or the *Yogacarya* about these visions, I am sure they intuitively understood. *Yogacarya* would invariably say something in the class that would help me put the visualization in perspective and derive a meaning out of it. This association between the *Yoga Sutra* and inner discoveries has been my constant companion till today. Though the classes have formally ended years ago, every time I encounter a different circumstance, meanings of a specific *Yoga Sutra* spontaneously echo in my mind and I find a way to deal with the situation. Since much of my work today is in listening to people and understanding group dynamics, these connections are direct. But, often, I find these echoes of immense help in other circumstances as well. I believe this is what *Yogacarya* meant when he talked about a "transfer of power" in the act of teaching. Each *sutra* he taught is embedded in me like a seed waiting to sprout and offer a meaningful suggestion in times of doubt and anguish.

I ask *Yogacarya* a doubt

One of the most lasting impressions I have of *Yogacarya* is the time I dared to ask him a doubt! The discipline of the class was clear. Until one had learnt and applied the learning without question, one had no basis to really ask questions! I have come to appreciate this discipline more and more as I teach others. The "modern" way that encourages debate and discussion is rather superficial. It is probably relevant in areas that are in the "measurable-logical" spectrum of experience. Unless one has tried to internalize the knowledge, the questions are invariably intellectual.

"What does *prana* mean? It is used in so many different ways in the various texts," I asked.

"I will answer this next week," was *Yogacarya*'s reply. Desikachar told me that *Yogacarya* went back to the texts and looked them up before answering me! The answer was two classes long! The depth of dedication to teaching and the sincerity of his commitment to a student left me profoundly touched and humbled.

Some time later, *Yogacarya* sustained a hip fracture and our classes with him stopped abruptly. A few months later, when he had recovered sufficiently, we went to pay our respects to him. *Yogacarya* asked me when we would resume classes since he had stopped the classes in the middle of the "*dahara vidya*" chapter of the *Chandogya Upanisad*. He recited the precise *sloka* that he had stopped at!

Epilogue

After close to ten years of intense study, practice, and teaching yoga at the KYM, I started focusing on my work with people and organisations in the area of Applied Behavioral Sciences. If one gets away from the notion that *asana* and *pranayama* encompass the entirety of yoga, one will understand that yoga as a study of inner transformation is profound and powerful. The *Yoga Sutra* that I learnt from *Yogacarya* and Desikachar forms the core of my work. By using the seminal ideas I have learnt from their teaching, and applying it to organizational problems, I have seen how universal and versatile the yoga of Krishnamacharya is. There is not a day that goes by when I do not remember him, or when one of the ideas he expounded in the classes does not come popping into my head. 〞

215

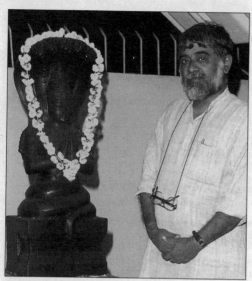

AV Balasubramaniam in front of Patanjali's statue.

AV Balasubramaniam

AV Balasubramanian is a scientist. He obtained his educational qualifications from some of the best institutions in the world, including the Indian Institute of Science, Bangalore, and State University of New York at Stonybrook. Since 1982, he has been involved in work relating to various aspects of Traditional Indian Sciences and Technologies, exploring their current relevance and potential. He met Krishnamacharya through Desikachar in the 1980s, and the relationship that developed between them has continued to impact his life. He is actively involved in many social projects and also in organic farming.

It was sometime during 1982, towards the end of the year, that I enrolled myself as a student at the Krishnamacharya Yoga Mandiram. After learning for four months, one day, I was asked to start teaching. I was pleasantly surprised but also quite nervous. Desikachar made light of my hesitation and cheerfully declared that teaching does not imply the end of learning, but, rather, that it is quite essential to even continue learning. It was thus that I started learning and also started attending the special sessions held for teachers.

One evening, towards the end of the teachers' class, Desikachar told us that he had received two visitors from the Hindu Mission Hospital. This hospital was a charitable institution. It had amongst its consultants some of the top medical specialists from the city of Madras. They requested Desikachar to depute a yoga teacher from the KYM to teach yoga to the patients at the hospital.

Desikachar posed the question at the teachers' meeting and added that the hospital authorities had wanted the yoga teacher to come on Sunday mornings. When there was no response from the teachers, Desikachar asked if he had to tell the hospital authorities that the KYM could not send a teacher on Sunday mornings. At this point, I offered to go to the Hindu Mission Hospital on Sundays. I immediately added a set of riders about how I would require a lot of help, guidance, and so on. Desikachar was very pleased, and in his usual manner, he waved aside all my reservations and congratulated me for offering to go on Sunday mornings.

When I went to the hospital, I found my first independent teaching assignment quite traumatic and trying. The first student I had was a sixteen-year-old boy, who was unable to eat any solids and had been on a liquid diet for several years. The second patient was a middle-aged lady, who had been unable to conceive, although both she and her spouse had been declared normal and medically fit for parenthood. The third case was that of a lady with a prolapsed uterus. I discussed the situation in detail with the students and gave them a course each, to the best of my knowledge and ability. I was told that the cases for which the hospital and the various specialists could offer no help had been told that there was a resident yoga expert whom they could consult for a possible cure. It is thus that I came to receive my first three students.

The next day, I told Desikachar the whole story. I told him that I would be very happy to teach yoga, but the kind of cases I had encountered were totally beyond my capacity, and that I felt completely out of my depth. He read through the case sheets and the courses that I had given and pondered over the matter for a few moments. He then said, "Let us go and consult my father." I was pleased and excited to hear this, since I had not yet met the legendary Krishnamacharya.

My first meeting

The next day, I went home with Desikachar to meet the *Yogacarya* [Krishnamacharya]. He had just suffered a small accident and fractured his hip. I went into the room and saluted him in the traditional manner. Desikachar told him in brief about my efforts and the students I had encountered. The *Yogacarya* asked us to describe a case, and I gave him the description of my first case, the boy who could not eat solid food. He pondered for a minute and asked, "Did they perform *Annaprasam* ceremony for this boy?" (*Annaprasam* is a traditional ceremony observed when an infant is given solid food for the first time). was quite startled and replied that I did not know. I had not thought of asking such a question. I answered in the negative, and he said that if I had to acquire the competence to treat such patients, I should have a basic knowledge of *Ayurveda* and certain rituals. We were silent for a while. Then Desikachar said, "Could you teach him and all of us by giving some lessons?"

The *Yogacarya* thought for a while and mentioned a date and time in the following week, when we could begin our lessons. I felt myself to be extraordinarily fortunate that I had thus got an opportunity to study directly with the *acarya*. Over the next year or two, he met a few of us regularly and shared a very valuable teaching.

During each meeting, he would spend an hour with us. He gave us introductory lessons on a wide range of subjects and would answer questions patiently. His manner was always soft and gentle and his comments, mild and encouraging. When I recited to him the problem of my first student, the boy who could not eat solid food and was constantly vomiting, he asked me what advice I had given and the course that had drawn up. I had given the boy a beginner's course and had also advised him to eat some tender neem leaves on an empty stomach every morning based on whatever limited knowledge I had of *Ayurveda* and home remedies. I had never imagined that this advice of mine and the course was going to be subject to a scrutiny by the *Yogacarya* himself. With great nervousness, I told him what I had prescribed. He was silent for a moment and then he looked at me, smiled and said, "*Paravalliye*," (roughly translates as "not bad at all"). I was pleased to hear such an endorsement of my course from the highest authority on the subject

I had always heard that words spoken by great saints and elders would come true even if they were said in jest. I feel this was indeed the case with Krishnamacharya. During our very first meeting, Desikachar introduced me to his father and said, "This is the person who is going to be the editor of our journal." A that time, we were planning to publish a journal from the KYM, which had been given the title "*Arogya Darsanam*," and preparations were in progress. On hearing these words of introduction, he spontaneously exclaimed, "But, he is so young!" I felt quite dismayed that the *yogacarya* had reacted thus, rather than giving his blessings and good wishes for the effort. As it turned out, his words proved to be prophetic. The journal that was planned in the '80s could not materialize and had to be abandoned. In 1991, it was given another try, and the Mandiram did indeed commence the publication of the journal—*Darsanam*—with myself as the editor. But, this time I was much older.

Learning from the *Guru*
One of the most important things that I believe I learnt from the *Yogacarya* was the meaning and significance of the *guru* and the methods of traditional healing. By any standards, Krishnamacharya was an outstanding teacher of yoga and a healer, and I believe that there are a lot of innovations and creative inputs that he has to his credit in many branches of ancient learning, particularly yoga.

However, it is striking to see that he would never proclaim anything as his own invention or even innovation. Whenever asked about the source of any knowledge or practice, he would invariable reply that he had obtained it from his *guru*. Initially, I had taken this to be a traditional proclamation of humility, and I missed the significance of his pronouncement. However, in the course of time, I could not but be struck by his astounding insights and creative interpretation of tradition in the modern context, and it gradually dawned on me that he was proclaiming what he saw as the pure truth in a very profound Indian way.

Krishnamacharya's teaching was always a very dynamic process. It was never merely the imparting of mere information or theories. He always used to proclaim, particularly in the context of teaching *mantras*, that when a *guru* teaches, he gives a part of his *sadhana* to his students. To Krishnamacharya, teaching a student was akin to the sowing of a seed. The tiny seed grows up to be a gigantic banyan tree, but it grows only if planted in fertile soil, and is nourished with water and light. If you cast the same seed on stone, you would not get a tree. One might pose the question, "Is the tree contained in the seed?" The tree is not contained in the seed in a trivial modern sense—if you cut it open, you cannot see small roots or branches or leaves within it. However, a tree is contained in the seed in the sense that the seed has the potential to mature and grow into a tree if it is nurtured over the years with water and light, and if it is raised in good soil. So also, it was considered that the *guru* who imparted knowledge planted the seed and was thus responsible for what it flowered into. After much thought, I came to the conclusion that it is in this sense that the *acarya* meant it, when he said that all his learning came from his *guru*.

Understanding the context of traditional knowledge

Krishnamacharya's learning was multifaceted, with knowledge of diverse disciplines such as *Nyaya, Veda, Vedanta, Mimamsa, Yoga, Ayurveda, Mantra*, music, etc., to name only a few. This gave him profound insights into the meaning and significance of our traditional practices and customs. For example, on one occasion, he was describing a ritual performed sitting in front of the sacred fire, and at one point he said that the narration on the *mantra* should stop and that one should get up and perform *pradaksina* (circumambulation) around the *agni* (fire) three times. Having said this, he said that for a person who was sitting cross-legged for one hour, to get up and do *pradaksina* was a proper *pratikriyasana* (counter pose). I was astonished at this observation. I had, of course, been taught the concept of *asana* and *pratikriyasana*, namely poses and counter poses in the context of yoga, where counterposes are performed to relieve any stress caused by the yogic postures. It was a revelation to me that the logic may also be used to analyze the meaning of certain rituals.

His humility was spontaneous and natural, and there was no affectation about him. I remember an incident where I had collected a large set of Tamil proverbs relating to home remedies for various problems and conditions, and we wanted his comments based on the *Sastric Ayurvedic* viewpoint. In several instances, he clearly stated that he could not comment on the practices whenever he had no basis for doing so. He would also clearly demarcate where his answers were based only on his reading, and other instances, where he had tested out the knowledge in practice.

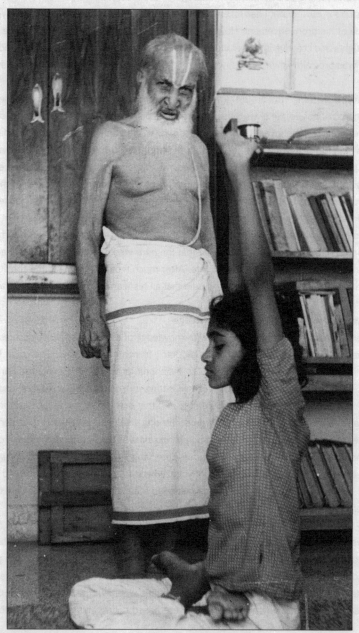

Krishnamacharya in his nineties, teaching a student.

He had the capacity to stay focused very clearly on the task at hand and would discourage questions that were asked merely to satisfy idle curiosity. I clearly remember an instance when he patiently heard me out—a set of questions at the end of which he asked a mild question—"What are we now trying to do?" After a pause, he himself answered, saying, "Let us first learn to be competent in those things that would be of direct benefit and immediate use for our people." I found this expression and words brought me back to reality with a thud from my exploration based on idle intellectual curiosity. I think his prescription is an excellent talisman for anyone who is trying to give direction to one's work.

I consider myself very fortunate that I met him at a time when he was gentle and mellowed. I had heard and read accounts of what a terror he was and how stern and tough he could be. My experience with him was so different that I must make a special mention of it. His manner was always gentle and unassuming, and he was very easily approachable. So far as I could see, he had a huge and varied procession of students throughout the day. They ranged from his very young grandchildren, his daughter-in-law, teachers of the Krishnamacharya Yoga Mandiram, Sanskrit scholars, industrialists, patients of all hues and colors with a range of problems, and also some of India's leading artistes, industrialists, and politicians.

My most vivid memory of him is his calm and beautiful smile. If I were to describe him in one word, I would choose the word *Bhakta,* or devotee, rather than a scholar, healer, or anything else. His faith in God was very deep and abiding. It was part of his being in a way that is very difficult to comprehend by someone who did not belong to his age and upbringing. I have heard on one occasion that an insurance salesman tried to sell him a policy and he was turned away with the matter-of-fact declaration, "Lord *Narayana* is my insurance. I need no other insurance." "

221

Besides his son, Krishnamacharya's three main students were Indra Devi, Pattabhi Jois, and BKS Iyengar. Indra Devi died in 2002, but her work is carried on through Fundacion Indra Devi. Pattabhi Jois died in 2009, and the Sri K. Pattabhi Jois Ashtanga Yoga Institute in Mysore currently continues his teaching under the direction of his grandson R. Sharath Jois and his daughter R. Saraswati. BKS Iyengar continues to teach at the center he founded in Pune.

Indra Devi

Fundacion Indra Devi

Azcuenaga 762.
Buenos aires (1029)
Argentina

phone: +54-11-4962-3112
fax: +54-11-4962-3112
e-mail: info@fundacion-indra-devi.org
website: www.fundacion-indra-devi.org

BKS Iyengar

Ramamani Iyengar Memorial Yoga Institute (RIMYI)

1107 B/1 Hare Krishna Mandir Road, Model Colony, Shivaji Nagar,
Pune, 411 015
Maharashtra, India

phone: +91-20-2565 6134
e-mail: info@bksiyengar.com
website: www.bksiyengar.com

Pattabhi Jois

Sri K. Pattabhi Jois Ashtanga Yoga Institute

#235, 8th Cross, 3rd Stage
Gokulam, Mysore 570002
Karnataka, India

phone: +91-9880185500
website: www.kpjayi.org